AUTOPHAGY

Discover your Self-Cleansing Body's Natural Intelligence, Heal your Body and Rapid Weight Loss through Alkaline Diet. Activate the Anti-Aging Process with Fasting and Water Benefits

Emma Medicine

© **Copyright 2019 by Emma Medicine - All rights reserved.**

This eBook is provided with the sole purpose of providing relevant information on a specific topic for which every reasonable effort has been made to ensure that it is both accurate and reasonable. Nevertheless, by purchasing this eBook you consent to the fact that the author, as well as the publisher, are in no way experts on the topics contained herein, regardless of any claims as such that may be made within. As such, any suggestions or recommendations that are made within are done so purely for entertainment value. It is recommended that you always consult a professional prior to undertaking any of the advice or techniques discussed within.

This is a legally binding declaration that is considered both valid and fair by both the Committee of Publishers Association and the American Bar Association and should be considered as legally binding within the United States.

The reproduction, transmission, and duplication of any of the content found herein, including any specific or extended information will be done as an illegal act regardless of the end form the information ultimately takes. This includes copied versions of the work physical, digital and audio unless express consent of the Publisher is provided beforehand. Any additional rights reserved.

Furthermore, the information that can be found within the pages described forthwith shall be considered both accurate and truthful when it comes to the recounting of facts. As such, any use, correct or incorrect, of the provided information will render the Publisher free of responsibility as to the actions taken outside of their direct purview. Regardless, there are zero scenarios where the original author or the Publisher can be deemed liable in any fashion for any damages or hardships that may result from any of the information discussed herein.

Additionally, the information in the following pages is intended only for informational purposes and should thus be thought of as universal. As befitting its nature, it is presented without assurance regarding its prolonged validity or interim quality. Trademarks that are mentioned are done without written consent and can in no way be considered an endorsement from the trademark holder.

Table Of Contents

Alkaline Diet

Introduction 1
Chapter 1 All about the Alkaline Diet 2
   What is the Alkaline Diet? 2
   Is the Alkaline Diet for You? 4
   What is pH? 5
   What is Alkalinity? 7
   Why is the Alkaline Diet so Important? 9
Chapter 2 Be Careful! 12
   How Food Affects Your Body 12
   What Can and can't be Affected by What You Eat? 14
   What Can the Alkaline Diet Prevent? 16
   We are What We Eat 21
Chapter 3 Our Health Leader, Microbiome 24
   What is the Microbiome? 24
   What is its Role in Alkalinity? 27
   Why it is Important? 28
   What is Autophagy? 30
Chapter 4 The Three Golden Keys- Reset, Rebalance, and Reconnect 32
   Reset 33
   Rebalance 35

Reconnect 39

How the Body Defends Itself 42

Chapter 5 Acid-Forming Foods and Habits to Avoid .. 46

Foods to Avoid 46

Habits to Avoid 49

Consequences of an Acid-Alkaline Imbalance 51

Chapter 6 Benefits of the Alkaline Diet 53

Physical Benefits 53

Mental Benefits 56

Emotional Benefits 57

Importance of Health 59

Chapter 7 Alkaline Foods to Enjoy 61

Alkaline Fruits 61

Alkaline Veggies 63

Other Alkaline Foods & Alkaline Water 66

Alkaline Meals 70

Chapter 8 Troubleshooting 72

The First Few Weeks 72

Cravings 75

Social Eating and Drinking 77

Portion Control and Getting Enough Nutrients 80

Chapter 9 Tips and Tricks 85

Ways to Maintain the Habit 85

v

Meal Prepping 87
An Overall Healthier You 88
Conclusion 91

Alkaline Diet Cookbook

Introduction 93

Chapter 1 What is the Alkaline Diet? 95

Chapter 2 The Benefits of the Alkaline Diet 104

Chapter 3 All about the Foods 116

Chapter 4 The 10-Day Meal Plan 125

Chapter 5 The Breakfast Recipes You Need 128

   Chia Parfait 128

   Warm Apple Pie Cereal 130

   Tofu Scramble 132

   Sweet Potato Parfait 134

   Tofu Morning Sandwich 135

   Nutty Overnight Oats 136

   Sunnyside Breakfast Bowl 138

   Breakfast Fruit Crepes 139

   Fruity Breakfast Salad 141

   Mocha Pudding 143

   Broccoli Omelet 144

   Tofu and Kale Tacos 145

   Savory Breakfast Bowl 146

   Almond Butter and Jelly Overnight Oats 147

Chapter 6 Easy Smoothie Recipes 149

   Tropical Smoothie 149

Ginger Smoothie 150

Vegetable Smoothie 152

Lime and Coconut Smoothie.. 153

Berry Blast Smoothie 154

Minty Morning Shake... 156

Fruit and Green Tea Smoothie 158

Apple Pie Smoothie... 159

Detox Juice 160

Fruity Lemonade..161

Chapter 7 Lunch Recipes 163

Southwest Stuffed Sweet Potatoes................................... 163

Zoodles with Cream Sauce 165

Rainbow Pad Thai... 167

Lentils and Greens 169

Sesame Greens Dish 170

Sweet Spinach Salad 171

Steamed Green Bowl 172

Vegetable and Berry Salad 173

Quinoa and Carrot Bowl.. 174

Grab and Go Wraps 177

Nutty Tacos 178

Tex-Mex Bowl 180

Avocado Soup and Salmon.. 182

Asian Pumpkin Salad 183

Sweet Potato Wraps 185

Spicy Cabbage Bowl 187

Citrus and Fennel Salad 189

Chapter 8 Dinner Recipes to Bring the Family Together 191

Vegetable and Salmon Kebabs 191

Coconut Curry with Vegetables 194

Loaded Spaghetti Squash 195

Spicy Pasta 196

Stuffed Peppers 198

Baba Ganoush Pasta 200

Cheesy Broccoli Bowl 202

Green Bean and Lentil Salad 203

Vegetable Minestrone 205

Southwest Burger 207

Zucchini Rolls with Red Sauce 209

Meatless Taco Wraps 211

Sesame and Quinoa Pilaf 214

Blackened Salmon with Fruit Salsa 216

Arugula Salad with Shrimp 218

Easy Pizza 221

Chapter 9 Snack Recipes for Easy Snacking 223

Watercress and Endive Boats 223

Toasted Trail mix 225

Avocado Chickpea Cups 226

Cocoa Truffles with Spice 228

Zesty Chips 228

Summer Fruit Soup 230

Maple Roasted Carrots 231

Smokey Caesar Salad 232

Spicy Mix with Tortilla Chips 233

Creamy Broccoli Soup 234

Tortilla Soup 236

Alkaline Gazpacho 237

Butternut Squash Soup 239

Chilled Tomato Soup 241

Baked Sweet Potato Fries with BBQ Sauce 243

Eggplant and Cashew Bites 245

Chapter 10 Dessert Recipes to End the Day 248

Cookie Dough Bites 248

Cashew Chip Cookies 250

Lemon Cookies 252

Lemon Lime Jelly 253

Strawberry Lime Bites 254

Coconut Chip Bites 255

Sweet Potato Orange Cookies 257

Cashew Cold Cookies 258

Pumpkin Cups 259

Apricot Crumble 260

Apricot Tarts 262

Raw Berry Crumble 264

Raspberry Cheesecakes 266

Chocolate Donut Holes 268

Banana and Oatmeal Cookies 270

Cinnamon Buns 271

Bonus Understanding the Use of Herbs in the Alkaline Diet 273

Conclusion 279

Alkaline Diet

A Beginner's Guide to Understanding PH, Eat Well and Boost Health Through Plant Based and Alkaline Foods for Bring your Body Back to Balance,Weight Loss and Heal Your Body Naturally.

Introduction

Perhaps you've tried diets before, but you haven't had any luck. You're looking for a way to switch it up and try something new. With the alkaline diet, you are using your body's pH levels to your benefit. In this book, you will learn the facts about the alkaline diet. You'll find out if it's the right diet for you, what the alkaline diet is, and all about pH. You will learn about the importance of the diet, as well as any considerations that you may need to make before starting it. You will also learn that you must be careful, as the food you put into your body greatly affects your health in many aspects. Further, microbiome and its role in alkalinity will be discussed, as well as the three golden keys (reset, rebalance, and reconnect). There are also certain foods and habits that you must avoid, as your body must be receiving the proper sources of energy and remain balanced. There are many benefits to the alkaline diet, as well as wonderful foods to enjoy. However, it is also important to be educated on the common mistakes that people make, as well as other tips and tricks for the diet. Overall, it is very important to be educated before starting a new diet. You must learn all about how food affects your body, as well as how to properly implement that diet. The alkaline diet is quite simple once you understand the concept of pH and alkalinity. However, you must be educated first to ensure that you are ready for the diet and are implementing it the proper way.

Chapter 1

All about the Alkaline Diet

Before jumping into the alkaline diet, you should be aware of what it is and how it will affect your body. The alkaline diet has been known to help with losing weight and preventing arthritis and cancer. Before beginning it, however, you must know how to do it, the science behind it, and any considerations you should make before committing to the diet. Your diet is extremely important for life. What you put in your body directly affects all of your functions. Your energy level, ability to sleep, and productivity are directly affected by your diet. By improving your diet, you are improving your ability to perform your everyday functions. You are also improving your long-term health, which is important for your future to ensure that you are healthy and live a long life.

What is the Alkaline Diet?

The alkaline diet consists of foods that are alkaline-promoting, such as fruits, vegetables, beans, tofu, nuts, seeds, and legumes. Foods that are not allowed in this diet are animal products (meat, dairy, and eggs) and processed foods (pre-packaged and canned foods). As far as drinks, water and pure juices are allowed. To enjoy the maximum benefits of this diet, alcohol, and caffeine should not be consumed. The alkaline diet has an emphasis on pure, whole foods. These foods are alkaline-promoting, as opposed to acidic. By using the science of pH, you can maximize your body's health and performance. Consuming the wrong foods can cause your body to produce acid. This is harmful to your body and can reduce the performance of your digestive and immune systems. Following the alkaline diet can also promote weight loss. In addition to reducing your body's acid production, you will be eating more pure foods. Reducing the amount of added sugars and unhealthy fats in your diet will greatly help with weight loss. To maximize the alkaline diet, you should completely cut out acid-producing foods. However, you can still experience the benefits by gradually reducing what you consume to alkaline-promoting foods. For example, cutting out acid-producing drinks (alcohol, soda, sugary juices, milk, etc.) and replacing them with water can make a massive difference in your life. You will be less fatigued, have more energy, experience weight loss, and be healthier overall. By gradually reducing the amount of acid-producing foods and increasing the amount of alkaline-promoting foods that you consume, you are doing your body a great favor. Overall, the alkaline diet consists of eating typical healthy foods. Reducing the processed foods in your diet and switching to pure foods (pure meat, vegetables, and fruits) is a step in the right direction and is typical for healthy diets. However, the alkaline diet takes it a bit further. Everything that you consume must be more alkaline-promoting food, as opposed to acidic food. This diet allows you to eat healthier and receive more proper nutrients. However, the alkaline diet may not be for everyone. There are some things that you must consider before you commit to the alkaline diet.

Is the Alkaline Diet for You?

Of course, before making drastic changes to your diet, there will be some aspects to take into consideration. It is not only a diet change but a lifestyle change. You must ensure that it is realistic for you and healthy for you. Before starting this diet, be sure that you talk to your doctor beforehand. If you have certain health conditions, it may not be the right diet for you. You may also consider partially committing to the alkaline diet. Instead of fully eating alkaline-promoting superfoods, you may opt for a more "hybrid" diet in which you eat some alkaline-promoting foods and some foods that are more acidic. This may also be helpful at first, as it may be a huge transition from your previous diet to completely cut out all acidic foods. Be sure that you ask your doctor about their opinions on whether the diet is right for you. That way, you can be safe and know if your body will be able to handle the diet. The doctor may be able to make further suggestions to you about the diet. Additionally, diets are a lot of work. It isn't easy to just completely switch what you eat. For some people, eating is fun and unhealthy foods bring them joy. If you are one of those people, it may be extremely difficult for you to cut out those foods from your diet so suddenly. You must also ensure that you don't "bounce back" on your diet. This means that you can't consistently eat well only to suddenly give up and lose all of your progress. It is something that you must stick with. This will require discipline. Eating truly is a social event. People typically drink alcohol at social events, yet the alkaline diet promotes the drinking of only water. Grabbing ice cream with family or friends will not be an easy task for you after starting the alkaline diet, as dairy is acidic food. You will have to resist the temptation of foods and drinks that are not alkaline-promoting.

After switching, you will most likely experience cravings of the old foods that you used to consume. You may face the social temptation to eat foods that are not allowed in the diet. You may have to drastically change the foods you buy at the store and eating out will be more difficult. This takes much motivation and discipline. However, if you are willing, it is possible. You must be able to recognize the importance of taking care of your body and eating well. If you place that above the temptations of acid-producing food, then you will be able to succeed. Overall, it will be difficult. You must consult a doctor prior to starting the diet. If you are motivated and your body will be able to handle the diet, however, it is fantastic. The hard work is certainly worth it, as you will feel so much better both physically and mentally. It is a great achievement to set a goal and be able to stick with it.

What is pH?

To better understand the alkaline diet and its effect on the body, you must understand what exactly pH is. Scientifically speaking, pH is the measure of how densely an object is concentrated with hydrogen ions. The higher the pH, the lower the concentration of $H+$ ions. Hydrogen ions and pH are inversely related. A lower pH means a higher concentration of hydrogen ions. The pH values range from 0 to 14. This is the scale that pH is measured in. The higher the pH, the more basic (or alkaline) the object. A lower pH is considered more acidic. A pH of exactly 7 is considered neutral. It's $H+$ and $OH-$ ions are balanced. Each increase in pH unit on the scale results in a difference of ten times the concentration of $H+$ ions. For example, a pH of 1 has a hydrogen ion concentration of .1M, whereas a pH of 2 has a hydrogen ion concentration of .01M. Anything with a pH above 7 is considered "basic" or "alkaline," and anything with a pH below 7 is considered "acidic."

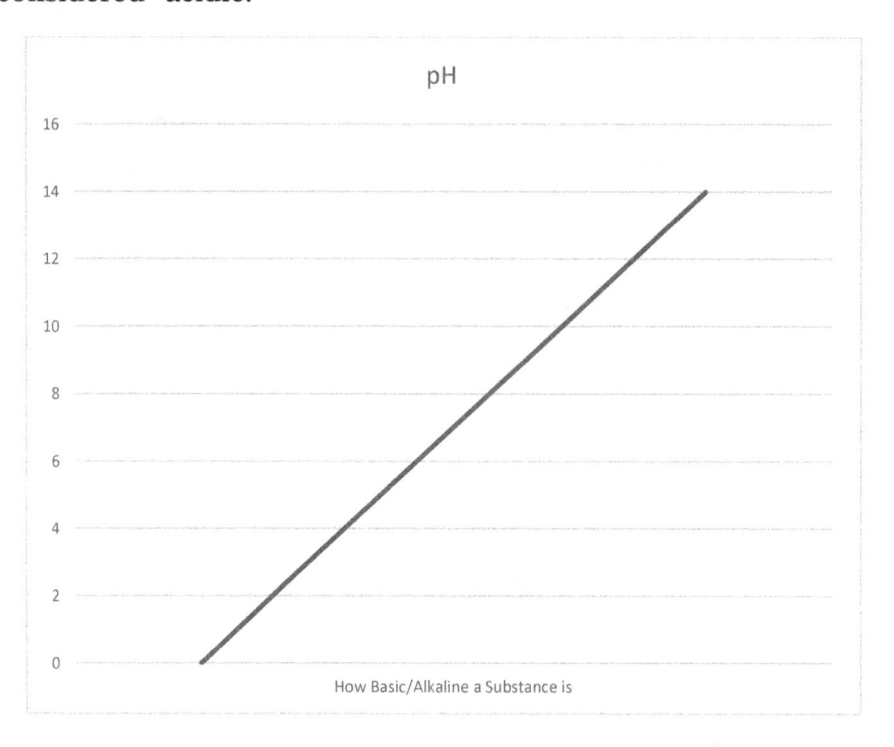

pH

How Basic/Alkaline a Substance is

Acids in foods release hydrogen ions and are therefore more sour-tasting. It is crucial to understand pH so that you may further understand your body and the way that food affects it. The pH of food affects the way that it can be handled. Depending on the pH of food, it may have to be prepared differently. Acidic foods only require boiling to be canned; this will effectively preserve the food. However, more basic foods may require the addition of citric acid to be safe and healthy for eating. The acidity helps to keep the food optimal for consumption. However, this is only for processed foods. Acidic foods are easier to preserve. With the alkaline diet, you will eat fresh foods and will not need to worry about this.

So, what are some real-world examples of foods on the pH scale? It is necessary to have points of reference to truly understand pH and how it works. First, you must understand that the truly neutral object, with a pH of 7, is pure water. Pure water (not bottled water, which contains additives) has a complete balance of H+ and OH- ions. Pure water is not realistic in the natural environment, as bottled, tap, and natural water contains traces of other elements. However, knowing that pure water has a pH of 7 is helpful. There are certain foods that lead to increased acidity in the human body, such as most grains, foods with added sugar, animal products, and sugary drinks. Lemon juice stands at a solid pH of 2, grapefruit is a 3, and tomatoes are around 4.6. Cabbage is a little over 5, mushrooms are about a 6. These are some of the few fruits and vegetables that have a higher acidity; however, fruits and vegetables tend to not have the negative, acid-producing effects of processed foods. Some more alkalizing foods are potatoes, beans, olive oil, and quinoa.

What is Alkalinity?

Alkalinity is the measurement of how many dissolved alkaline substances there are in a solution, and how well that solution is able to neutralize the acid. Depending on the pH, there will be a different type of alkalinity present. The three main types are bicarbonate, carbonate, and hydroxide. At around 4.3 pH, alkalinity occurs (anything from 0 to under 4.3 is purely carbon dioxide that is dissolved in the solution). At around 4.3, bicarbonate ions are present. At around 8.3, carbonate ions are present. At around 12, hydroxides are present. Alkalinity neutralizes acids, which balance the pH and make it more stable. This occurs by the addition or absorption of an H+ ion.

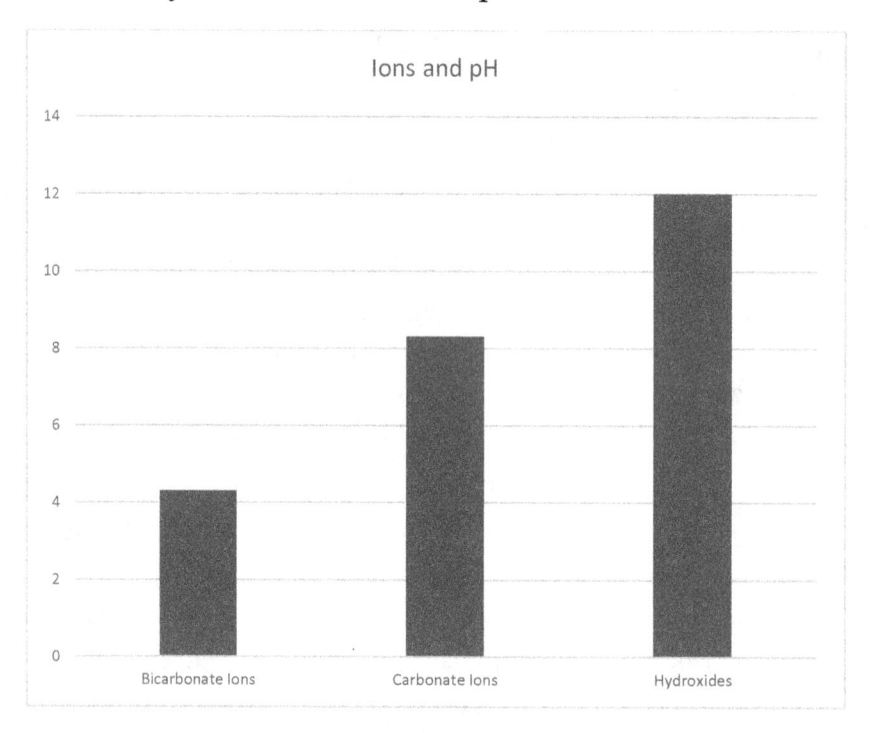

Ions and pH

Ion	Value
Bicarbonate Ions	~4
Carbonate Ions	~8
Hydroxides	12

Although pH and alkalinity are commonly confused, they are different. Whereas pH is the measure of the power of hydrogen ions, alkalinity measures the concentration of acid/alkali in the water. Higher alkalinity makes for a lesser chance of pH change. When the alkalinity is higher, the solution is more balanced and has a greater ability to neutralize the acid. Due to this, it is harder to lower the pH, as the solution will just neutralize any acidity that will occur in it.

Why is the Alkaline Diet so Important?

It is important that the body maintains a more alkaline environment. The greater the alkalinity, the harder it is to change the pH. If your body is more alkaline, then it will be more resistant to the buildup of acids in the body. This will also help your body maintain its functions. The body will have a better metabolism, which means that it will be able to break down food faster. This will allow for weight loss (or the maintenance of healthy body weight), a greater amount of energy, and an overall better ability to break down food. It will also allow for a better-functioning immune system. Because the body is able to function better, the immune system will also be able to work better. This means that the body can fight sickness better. With a better diet and environment for the body, you are allowing it to perform at its best. Your body will be able to defend you from any sickness that attempts to invade it much more effectively. This will result in fewer sicknesses in the first place. It also means that, if you do get sick, it will take less time to recover, as your body is able to better defend itself. Additionally, your body will be able to repair itself more quickly. Because the body has a better environment and is able to function better, it will be able to work harder to keep you at your healthiest. When you get injured, your body will be able to more quickly repair the damage that has been done. As a result of these, you will also see yourself performing better in day-to-day life. You will have more energy, will be less sick and recover more quickly from sickness, and will be able to repair yourself better when anything does go wrong.

The alkaline diet just makes sense. Your body has a natural internal pH of around 7.0. Because humans are composed of around 60% water, this makes perfect sense. For these reasons, water is highly stressed, as it greatly helps our bodies to function the way they are supposed to. When the body is maintained around this pH, it performs the way it is supposed to. Over time, humans have developed a tendency to consume more acidic foods. This proves detrimental to the body and its ability to function at its fullest capacity. When the body's internal environment fluctuates from being around 7.0, it becomes more difficult for the body to regulate itself. Having alkaline reserves will allow the body to be able to regulate the internal pH more efficiently and effectively. Because the body is constantly changing and having to adjust to the external environment, it is important to have as much internal stability as possible. Acid-forming foods lead to stress and inflammation of the body, which can cause a loss of energy and body bloat that presents itself in extra fat. By eating the proper foods, the body will be able to counteract any acids more effectively and be able to maintain the internal pH of the body.

Foods that are effective at forming alkaline include most fruits and vegetables. The alkaline diet stresses the consumption of these foods, and they compose a good amount of the diet. This is great because, in addition to regulating the body's pH levels effectively, these serve as powerful foods that are also healthy in other respects. They are packed full of vitamins and minerals that help your body to function the best that it can. They are also wonderful for increasing energy in a natural way. Instead of being loaded with added sugar, sodium, and fat, these foods are whole and natural. They keep your body energized.

An alkaline diet is also important for keeping your blood healthy and preventing high blood pressure. Because the blood's pH stays at around 7.0 to 7.5, regulating the body's pH and consuming alkaline-promoting foods is crucial. As your pulse is required for you to live, making sure that your blood is at its healthiest is very important to prevent problems with the heart, blood, and general circulation. When switching to an alkaline diet, you are ensuring that your body and its blood are healthier.

Further, an alkaline diet is crucial for your digestive health. Alkaline helps to promote healthy bacteria growth, which allows for better-functioning intestines. This means that your food can be digested well. Additionally, alkaline foods promote the repair of intestinal walls. As a result, any acid that gets in the body will be able to be counteracted, and the intestines will be able to be repaired from any damages. Furthermore, alkaline helps to suppress pathogen growth, leading to better digestive health.

Overall, an alkaline diet proves to help with the general health of the body. Regulating pH and alkalinity in the body is crucial for ensuring proper health.

Chapter 2

Be Careful!

How Food Affects Your Body

It's no secret; your diet affects your health. Your diet can affect your weight. It can affect your risk of heart disease, stroke, and diabetes. It can improve your immune system, digestive system, and cardiovascular health. With the alkaline diet, you are maximizing the benefits of eating healthy. You will live a longer and healthier life. Whereas those with diets composed of processed foods, sugary drinks, and acidic foods are putting themselves at risk for disease and obesity, those who follow the alkaline diet are actually preventing harmful processes from occurring in their bodies. A proper diet will also help you to have energy so that you may do all the activities that you want to do. You won't feel worn out constantly. On the flip side, eating acidic foods can bring you down. You won't have energy and will constantly feel tired. You will also feel hungry constantly, so you will want to put even more junk in your body and perpetuate this lethargic feeling.

By eating healthy, you are also allowing your body to maximize the nutrients that it receives. You're decreasing the amount of added sugar and sodium and sticking to the basics. Long before humans had factories that made pre-packaged snacks, fast food restaurants that cranked out an abundance of food, and grocery stores that offered around 35,000 different types of food options, they stuck to the basics, gathering all of the foods that they ate. This is what the human body was evolved into consuming. Berries, nuts, and such were the primary foods that were eaten by humans. This is what the human body is used to. Surprisingly, the human body is not made to process milk from cows. It is not natural. Yet, we consume dairy so frequently. We were certainly not made to eat greasy and salty French fries. These foods will not allow our bodies to receive the nutrients that they are supposed to, so it is no wonder that so many experience health problems. However, fixing your diet is an easy solution to this.

It is no surprise that a person's diet affects them greatly. After all, food is what we consume each and every day. It is necessary for our survival. It is the way that we obtain our energy. So why do most people tend to not care about what they put in their bodies? That shall remain a mystery. But once you recognize how important food is and how greatly it affects your body, it will be a no-brainer to put the proper foods in your body. If you consume an improper diet, you will become deficient in certain vitamins and minerals. The human body is all about balance and getting enough of what it needs. Much like how you won't be able to function well without a proper amount of sleep, you won't be able to properly function without receiving all of the proper nutrients. Your immune system won't be as strong, you won't have as much energy, and you will just feel unhealthy overall. When eating a proper diet, you also help your heart health. This is crucial. Your pulse is what keeps you alive. You can die from heart attacks and other heart issues that may arise. This is why it is so important for you to take care of your heart health. Your blood pressure and cholesterol will be maintained by eating a proper diet, which ensures that you are able to function well and have a healthy heart. Additionally, you will be able to have healthier and stronger bones and teeth, allowing you to move properly and reverse the process of aging in the bones. By eating properly, you are also ensuring that your weight stays down. If all you consume are cheeseburgers, fries, and soda, then it makes perfect sense that you will be overweight (or even obese). By maintaining your diet, however, you can prevent much of this from occurring.

What Can and can't be Affected by What You Eat?

Although you can greatly improve your health by improving your diet, you can't fix everything with a proper diet. With your weight, diet plays a huge role but it isn't the only factor. Getting enough exercise is important to ensure that you are the proper weight. Eating well will get your weight down, but if you don't get any exercise, you will not be in shape and will still lack strength in your muscles and bones. This is why a proper diet-exercise balance is necessary for your health. Also, if you don't go outside, you will not be the healthiest possible. Your body needs vitamin D, which it gets from the sun. Although you can get this from food, it is still important to get outside to ensure that you are getting fresh air and are getting some sunlight. Spending time outside has proven to improve blood pressure, help mental health, and lower the risk of cancer. Related to this is your environment. Your environment influences your health. With urban areas comes an increase in pollution. If you live in an area that is heavily polluted, the air quality will be lower. This can't be fixed by fixing your diet. You will suffer respiratory problems even if your diet is perfect. If you live in a place with a higher altitude, you may experience nosebleeds, dizziness, and respiratory issues. This may be helped by eating properly but may not be completely cured by a switch of diet. Additionally, the effects of smoking can't be changed by your diet. The risk for heart attack and lung disease is increased by smoking, and eating won't change that.

Furthermore, genetics plays a huge role in your health. If there are health problems that run in your family, then your risk for these issues is automatically increased. Although you can do your best to eat well, you will still always be at risk for these issues. You may decrease your risk, but there is still the possibility that you may develop problems. For instance, some people naturally possess a less efficient metabolism, and being overweight is a common problem in their family. Although you can regulate your diet and exercise to reverse this problem, it may always be easier for your body to gain weight, and you must be careful to monitor that. Certain races also have a higher risk of heart disease, which occurs naturally. This can't be changed, but you can do your best to take care of yourself and try to decrease your risk for these health issues. Gender also contributes to health problems. Women experience more deadly heart issues, yet men are diagnosed with heart issues more frequently. Hormones may also affect you. For instance, menstruation and menopause may not be prevented by eating well. However, a proper diet can make these processes smoother. Cramps caused by menstruation can be lessened with a reduction of dairy. Menopause is a natural occurrence that comes with aging. Aging is another factor that can't be changed. As you grow older, your body will naturally lose some of its health. Your risk for illness and disease increases, and it is harder for your body to operate the way that it used to.

In addition to the physical aspects affecting you and your health, mental health plays a massive role in your health. If you have strained relationships, you are likely to be stressed, anxious, and overall uneasy. This can lead to a plethora of problems. You can feel fatigued, in pain, have an upset stomach, and have trouble sleeping (in addition to many other health problems). It is important to maintain mental health. To prevent stress, it is important to get proper exercise, keep your space decluttered, maintain healthy relationships (and cut off those who aren't healthy to be around), take time to yourself, and do what makes you happy. Getting outside and having hobbies are important as well. Diet can only do so much for your health. Although diet can indirectly affect your health (it can give you more energy to be active, which subsequently lowers your stress), you must ensure that other aspects of your body remain healthy. The body is composed of many systems that work together. When one system isn't taken care of or stops working properly, everything else is affected. This is why it's so important to care for your health in many aspects. Although diet plays a massive role in your overall health, it isn't the only aspect of your health that you must care for.

What Can the Alkaline Diet Prevent?

The alkaline diet serves as a very healthy diet and can lead to a number of benefits for your health. In addition to helping to regulate your body's pH, there are other reasons why this helps your body to be healthier and function better. The alkaline diet puts a heavy focus on eating the right foods for your body. It emphasizes a diet consisting of fruits and vegetables, as well as water. Processed foods and sugary drinks are eliminated from one's diet. By cutting out harmful foods and instead consuming healthy foods, you are keeping your bones and muscles strong. This can reduce the effects of osteoporosis that occur with aging, as well as other muscle and bone issues from arising. This will also decrease pain, as the bones and muscles will be healthier. They will also repair and recover more easily, as the environment in the body is more optimal for functioning. This will help you to stay healthier and remain active. There is also improved cardiovascular health, which can prevent heart disease. A better diet also allows for lower blood pressure and lower cholesterol, which further helps heart health. Mental health will be improved, as you will be able to think more clearly and have more energy. You will feel less stressed as well.

The alkaline diet is well-known for its "cancer-curing" powers. Although the alkaline diet can help to decrease your chances of developing cancer and even make the treatment process easier and quicker, it can't completely cut out any possibility of cancer. However, it can help to lower your risk of it. It has been found that cancer cells thrive in more acidic environments. As a result, establishing a more alkaline environment in your body can help to decrease the likelihood of these cells growing in your body. Although there's no real way to alter the pH of your blood (as it is regulated by the lungs and kidneys), you can slightly change the pH of your saliva and urine quite easily. The foods also affect your body because they are better for you. It can help you to feel your best and your body to work at its best. This will help you to lower your risk of cancer and to treat it faster if you develop it.

The alkaline diet can also prevent obesity. Because your diet will be plant-based and lacking processed foods, you will be living without all of the added sugar and sodium that turn into fat in the body. This means that you will be able to lose weight and keep that weight off if you stick with the diet. Because fruits and vegetables are less densely concentrated in calories, you will have to eat much more to have the same caloric intake. Whereas one common fast-food burger contains over 300 calories, you would have to eat three whole apples to consume around 285 calories. This makes you more conscious of what you're eating. Instead of quickly shoving a pre-packaged snack in your mouth, you can actually enjoy the eating experience.

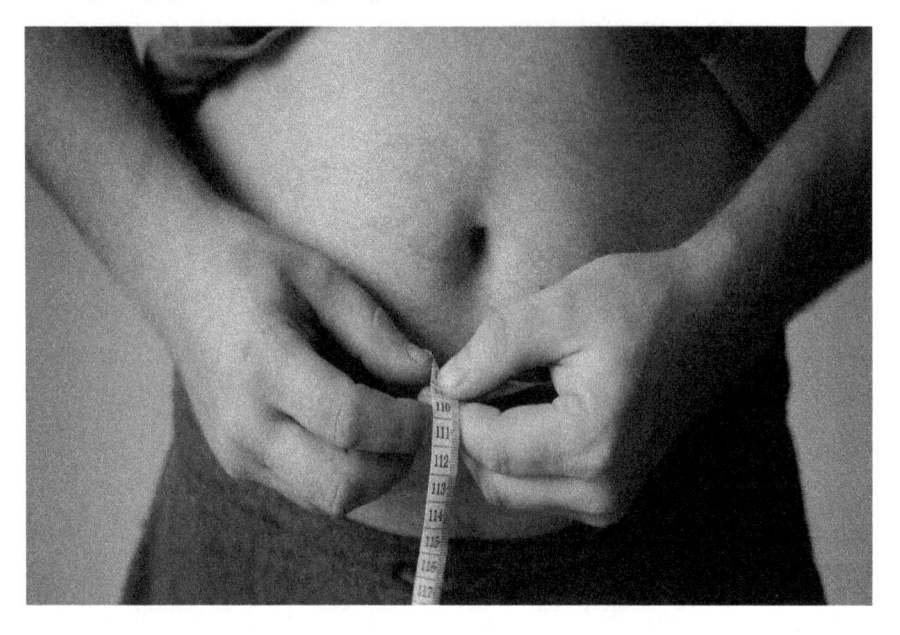

Additionally, the alkaline diet places a heavy focus on drinking water. Drinks such as juices and sodas typically contain a large amount of added sugar. They also lead to an assortment of health problems. By drinking water, you are keeping your body much healthier. One health problem that you are preventing is kidney stones. These occur when urine contains crystal-forming substances and your kidney develops "stones." These are very painful and should be prevented when possible. By drinking water, cutting out unneeded sugar and salt, and not eating an excess of protein, you can keep your kidneys healthy and prevent kidney stones from forming in the first place.

Another health issue that the alkaline diet can help to prevent is hypertension. This is also known as high blood pressure. High blood pressure can lead to an increased risk of heart disease, stroke, and even death. As a result, the prevention of high blood pressure is extremely important. Blood pressure is how much force is put upon your blood vessel walls by your blood. When too much pressure is applied, high blood pressure results. An excess of sodium in one's diet can contribute to this problem, and this can be prevented by cutting out the amount of salt in one's diet.

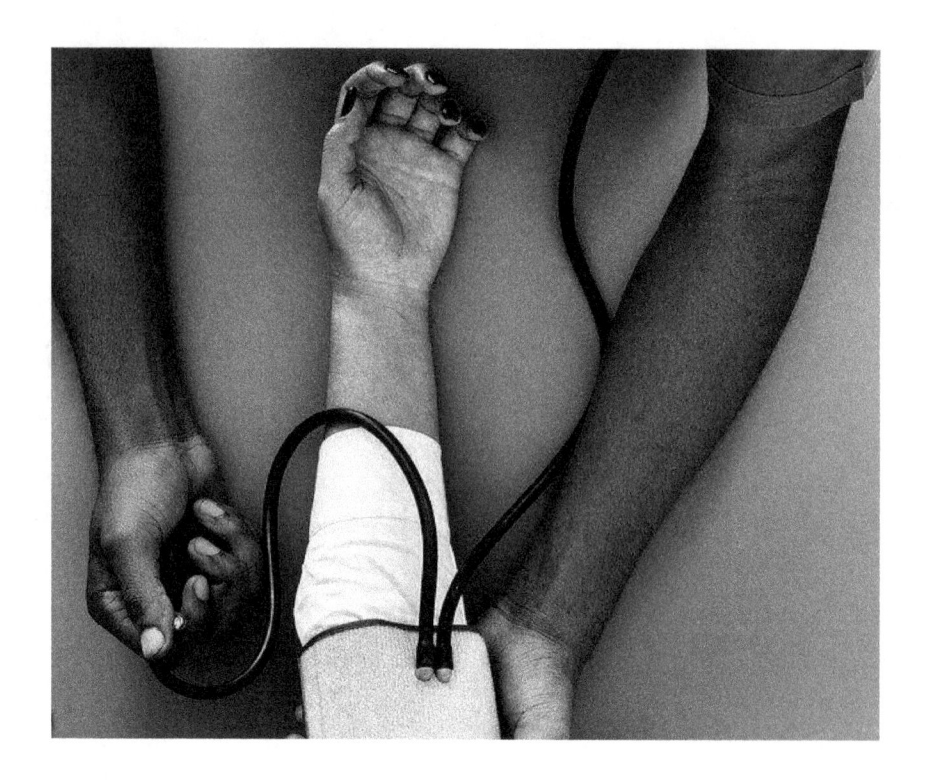

Processed foods, and especially foods made at restaurants, contain a great excess of salt. This is typically added to enhance the flavor of foods. However, it is not worth the health problems that accompany it. The alkaline diet focuses on fruits and vegetables, which are natural and don't contain any addition of sodium. They can also be delicious, so salt and sugar are not needed to enhance the naturally delicious foods that they are.

The alkaline diet is amazing for preventing health problems. The decreased risk of health issues can help to allow you to live a longer and healthier life. You will also feel better performing day-to-day functions, as your body will be able to function more efficiently and effectively.

We are What We Eat

It is important to avoid junk foods, as they contribute to a variety of health problems. It is very tempting to eat junk food. There is social pressure, as a common social activity is to go to a restaurant with friends and family while enjoying being served food. It is fast and convenient to open up a pre-made snack, pop a frozen meal in the microwave, or pull up at the drive-thru of a fast food restaurant. It is also cheap. Because those foods are mostly a bunch of chemicals and preservatives that are thrown together and mass-produced, they are cheap to make and therefore inexpensive to buy. However, the phrase "you are what you eat" is very true. If you put junk into your body, your health will reflect that. If you eat well, you will feel much better and your body will be much healthier. Junk food causes a variety of problems in the body.

Food that is high in sodium increases your risk of developing headaches. These can be painful, irritating, and prevent you from being able to focus. An excess of sodium can also lead to hypertension (high blood pressure). It can also cause your body to be bloated and "puffy." Junk food can also cause acne, as carbohydrates are not healthy for your skin. An excess of sugar can lead to poor dental health. Processed foods can lead to weight gain, which can result in obesity and shortness of breath, as well as an increased difficulty to remain active. It can also lead to heart disease and stroke. Fast food leads to poor blood sugar levels, which can increase your risk of type-2 diabetes. Consuming Tran's fats can lead to high cholesterol. These sorts of foods can also damage your digestive system and prevent it from functioning at its fullest potential. Your body won't be able to break down these foods as easily, and your pancreas will suffer as a result of the sugar excess. When you gain weight, your respiratory system will suffer. There will be added stress to your heart and lungs, and it will be harder to breathe, especially while in motion. The reproductive system will also suffer and eating junk food may even lead to an increased risk of infertility and birth defects. Your body's skeletal and muscular systems will suffer. In addition to the added stress put on your body by an excess of fat, you will also be lacking vital nutrients and vitamins that help strengthen your body. Your appearance will also suffer. Junk food will lead to acne, poor hair health, unhealthy nails, and can increase your risk of eczema. Not only will you feel unhealthy, but your appearance will reflect that as well.

In addition to negative physical effects on your body, junk food can decrease your mental health. Your mental health will indirectly and directly be affected by this food. You may feel worse mentally because you are self-conscious of your body and feel guilty about what you eat. Junk food has also been shown to decrease energy, which may leave you feeling unmotivated and not as active. This will also make you feel bad. Junk food also increases your risk of depression. This is both because the food is unhealthy for your brain's health and because you lack the energy and motivation that healthier foods give you. An unhealthy diet is also a cause of dementia, as blood pressure and cholesterol levels are high. The brain, as a result, will only be able to function poorly. Junk food also leads to stress, which can cause further problems (such as lack of sleep, stomach issues, etc.). Junk food also causes blood sugar levels to be unhealthy, which can lead to confusion and impair the thinking process.

The alkaline diet is important for your health. Although it can't cure every problem out there, it can prevent a number of health issues from arising and decrease your risk of many health problems. You can live longer with a better diet, and you can be able to enjoy life more if you eat properly. The alkaline diet truly affects your body and it is extremely important to ensure that your body is functioning at its best.

Chapter 3

Our Health Leader, Microbiome

What is the Microbiome?

Microbes (short for microscopic organisms) are living creatures that are too small to be seen without a microscope. This general category for living organisms encompasses several types of life-forms, which include bacteria, fungi, viruses, and other microscopic organisms. In the human body, there are many microbes, and many types of microbes. Although bacteria and microscopic creatures have bad reputations and are seen as things that cause sickness, this isn't always the case. Most bacteria that are in the body are actually beneficial. For instance, there are many bacteria that work to help your body to digest food properly. Without these creatures helping you out, your body would be unable to function properly. There are only certain types of bacteria that are harmful to you. Bacteria are very diverse. Archaea, another type of microbe, can live in extreme environments and have a special membrane that surrounds them. Fungi are important in decomposition. They are able to break down organisms and obtain nutrients from them; however, there are many harmless fungi that live on the human body. Protists are diverse but are sometimes the cause of diseases. There are also many harmless and even beneficial protists that live in the human body. Viruses infect the hosts. They usually target a certain cell type within the host. They may even infect other microbes within the host's body. Microscopic animals live on bodies and are usually harmless and aren't noticed by the one they dwell on. Microscopic plants serve as a source of energy for animals and release oxygen.

The microbiome means all of the microbes in a community. In this context, it means all of the microbes in the human body. They live in our bodies, especially in the intestines, mouth, and reproductive system. They also live on the outside of the body on the skin and in hair. This community of trillions of microbes serves as an important regulator of human health for the body. The microbiome also means the collection of genes of all of the human body's microbes. The microbiome is important in human health. If kept healthy, the microbes will serve a beneficial role in the body's functioning. Microbes help with the immune and digestive systems especially. The microbiome is constantly changing. Outside factors heavily contribute to the body's microbiome. This is why it is important to take care of your body and have the proper diet to ensure that your body is the healthiest that it can be.

The microbiome is present everywhere. The human body has its own microbiome, but every environment is home to microbes. Throughout the early years of development, humans accumulate microbes to add to their microbiome. The first three years of a human's development are the most important years for the microbiome. These years are composed of the mass collection of these organisms, which are beneficial for the body and essential for life. Humans collect a great variety of microbes to add to their grand microbiome. There are many microbes that have developed the ability to live in extreme conditions, and they can be found everywhere as a result. From the deepest parts of the ocean to the tallest points of mountains, there will be microbes. There are, of course, different types that will live in different areas. However, a huge variety of microbes live inside of our bodies. They play a massive role in the function and health of our bodies. It is important to have such a variety in and on the body, as each microbe serves a specific role in the body. Without microbes, we wouldn't be able to function as well as we do. In fact, we would not be able to live. Microbes are incredibly crucial. They help us to function in ways that the body wouldn't be able to do alone. This is why it's so important to understand the microbiome, the role it plays, and how to keep it healthy.

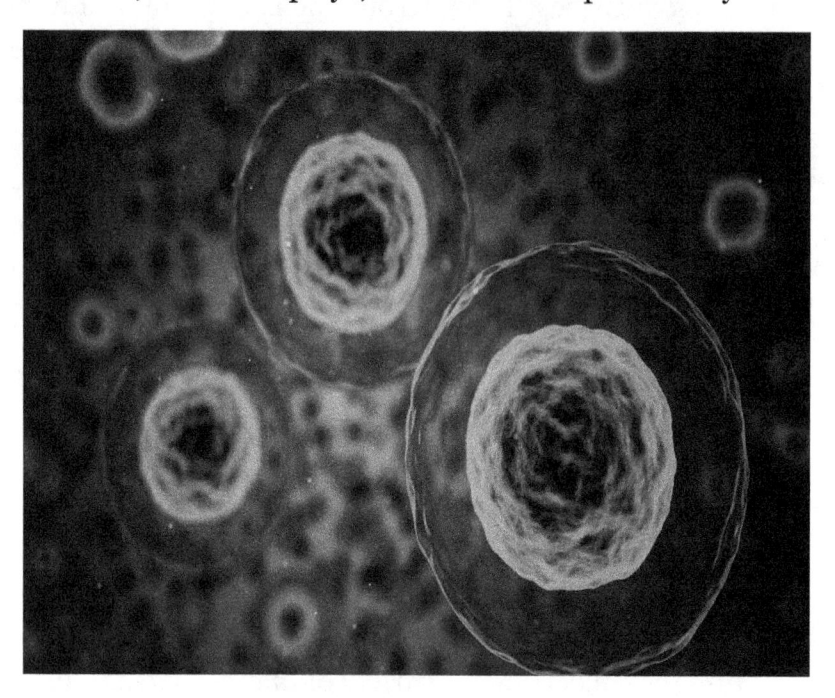

What is its Role in Alkalinity?

Research has been conducted on the role of pH on the body's microbiome. It has been concluded that consuming more acidic water leads to increased development and progression of diseases in the body. It greatly affects the diversity of microbes in the gut, which is crucial to the ability to digest food properly. With a decreased diversity of microbes comes the decrease of beneficial microbes that help to prevent and fight disease. So, not only will the body struggle to digest food, but it will also struggle to fight disease. Overall, a lower pH is shown to have a negative effect on the microbiome. This is very important to know. Knowing this, it makes sense that we must keep our pH more alkaline. Otherwise, we risk losing the variety of beneficial and harmless microbes in our bodies that are helping our bodies function the proper way. Reducing the alkalinity will disallow the body to neutralize the acids in the body, leading to a further decrease in the internal pH of the body. This leads to even further deterioration of the microbes within the body. Essentially, having a more acidic diet leads to a chain reaction of unhealthiness. The alkaline diet is important to allow the body's microbiome to function properly. Your body, as a result, will be able to digest properly, prevent and defend against diseases better, and be overall healthier. You lower your risk of illnesses, diseases, and conditions that will hurt your health. Acids disallow bacteria to grow. This is why many processed foods are more acidic. This preserves them for longer and disallows bacteria to grow inside of them. While that may be helpful for food, bacteria are beneficial for the body and are necessary for your body to function properly. It is best to avoid acidic foods and maintain a more neutral pH in your body so that your microbiome is healthy and functioning well. Although it may seem like it will be harder for harmful bacteria to grow in your body when the pH is lower, which is true, this is not beneficial overall. Although you're decreasing the number of harmful bacteria, you are also decreasing the number of beneficial bacteria that would be able to defend your body against such microbes. If external microbes that are harmful are introduced to your body, you will be lacking the proper defense system for keeping yourself healthy. This is why the alkaline diet is so important for your health.

Why it is Important?

The microbiome is very important because microbes make up a great amount of our body. In fact, there are ten microbes for each human cell in your body. In the gut alone, humans can have over 1,000 different species of bacteria that live and work with the body. The primary function of bacteria in the body is to help the immune and digestive systems, and the majority of bacteria in the human body lives in the intestines. Microbes are also important for the immune system, as they help the body defend itself from any sickness and potential invasions to the immune system. They also help to break down foods that may be otherwise toxic to the body. They break down foods that are otherwise difficult for the body to digest. This is why the many microbes in the large intestine are so important. By eating the proper foods and regulating your microbiome properly, you are ensuring that you are able to stay the healthiest that you can be.

Without a healthy microbiome, there are health risks. You may not be able to regulate digestion and waste properly. Irritable bowel syndrome can result from an improper diet. Type 1 diabetes may also result from improper diet. With a healthy microbiome, you are also allowing your body to properly defend you from diseases, including deadly diseases. You are also lowering the risk of arthritis, multiple sclerosis, and fibromyalgia. Consuming the proper foods is crucial for your health, and even for your survival. Diet affects so much of our bodies. It plays a central role in our microbiome's health, which affects many aspects of our body and its functions. By eating a healthy diet, you are ensuring that the microbes in the colon are proper. One factor that affects this is how much fiber is in your diet. With higher fiber and a subsequent lower pH, there is a lower amount of growth of certain bacteria. Foods that contain prebiotics (most fruits, vegetables, and beans) are great for feeding the beneficial bacteria in our bodies.

The microbiome also helps to produce vitamins that are essential for human health. Without the health of the microbiome, you risk malnutrition and the dysfunction of the human body. Microbes also contain 200 times the amount of genetic material than the human genome. They also help with human development and are especially important in the early years of life. The fact that they can adjust to a number of conditions shows how important diet is to health. With even the slightest fluctuation, microbes will adjust. They aren't stationary; they are constantly changing. This is why we must ensure that we are providing them with the most optimal conditions possible. Although there are some factors that we have little to no control over, such as the external environment that surrounds us or diseases that are currently spreading, there is one thing that we have great control over diet. With a proper diet, you are allowing the microbes in your body to perform at their best and also allowing you to live the healthiest life that you can. Most microbes are either harmless or beneficial. If you treat them well and give them what they need to remain healthy, they will, in turn, keep you healthy. It is important that they stay balanced and are living in the most optimal environment for them.

What is Autophagy?

Autophagy is the process of natural regeneration that occurs in the body at the microscopic level. This regeneration of cells leads to a decrease in the chance of diseases. It will also increase the body's lifespan. It's been proven that fasting stimulates autophagy, but doctors have yet to come up with the exact times for fasting. Coupling fasting with the alkaline diet can maximize the benefits of autophagy and allow the body to experience a great amount of cellular regeneration. Autophagy allows cells to be renewed and supplies the body with energy. It can also help the immune system to defend the body against harmful bacteria and viruses. It can also work to counteract aging and lead to a longer lifespan. It also helps the mind and memory. Overall, autophagy can really help a person's health and should be maximized as much as possible. Diet can play a role in enhancing this process. The alkaline diet can stimulate a better environment for the body and lead to a subsequent increase in the efficiency and effectiveness of autophagy. Autophagy allows the body to rid itself of old cells. Much like exfoliating the skin removes the dead skin cells and leaves a "clean slate," autophagy helps to rid the body of the old cells that it no longer needs and to turn those cells into new or renewed cells. The body essentially "eats" the old cells and turns them into new and fresh cells that can function at their fullest potential. It also allows your body to use what it already has to develop into something new and maintain the cleanliness of your body. It further allows your body to adjust to the environment and any toxins that may enter our bodies. This is important for your health. If autophagy is perfected, it can greatly increase the length of our lives, as is serves the function of anti-aging. Your body is creating "younger" cells by recycling the "older" ones. Short-term fasting serves as a way to force your body to undergo autophagy, as it must find a way to generate energy from what it already has. Autophagy may prevent cancer, diseases, and quick aging. The prevention of these is extremely important. The alkaline diet can work to improve the process of autophagy in the body.

The human body's microbiome is very powerful. If we are able to use that to our advantage, we may reap the benefits of the microbes that are working for us. To do that, however, we must take care of our body and its internal environment. The alkaline diet can do this, as it regulates our body's pH and allows for an improved internal environment. With this, the microbes inside of us are able to function better and keep us healthy. Autophagy is another process that really improves our health and should be utilized the most it can be to ensure that we are living the healthiest lives that we can be.

Chapter 4

The Three Golden Keys- Reset, Rebalance, and Reconnect

The alkaline diet will help you do the three golden keys: reset, rebalance, and reconnect. Because you were previously on foods that were less optimal, it is important that you are able to reset your body so that it is able to be healthy and functioning well. When consuming junk, you must reset, rebalance, and reconnect your body often. This is commonly done by "juicing," or drinking juices and smoothies that are made up of healthier foods. This will help your body to rid itself of any toxins and to establish better habits. You will feel better. It is also common to lose weight during these "reset" periods, as they are allowing your body to establish good habits and only eat foods that are beneficial for it. Although having reset/rebalance/reconnect periods are important for your body when eating junk food, they are unnecessary when starting the alkaline diet. This is because every day serves as a day to reset, rebalance, and reconnect your body. When you are eating the right foods, your body won't need a "break" from the junk. You'll be eating the proper foods each and every day.

Reset

The typical "detox" consists of resetting your body. Resetting your body is necessary for optimizing your health. Resetting your body is especially important if you have begun to feel lethargic and need some energy. Our bodies sometimes get worn down from stress, caffeine, or extra junk (especially around holidays and such). This makes resetting your body necessary. When starting the alkaline diet, you won't need weekly or monthly resets. Your body will be reset by the diet. You won't struggle with the side effects of caffeine (headaches, exhaustion, etc.) because you won't be consuming it any longer. When drinking only water, you are already resetting your body. Instead of drinking beverages with added sugar, caffeine, or alcohol, you are drinking what the human body craves naturally. This will help you to feel much better. Additionally, you will now be eating a plant-based diet, which is full of foods that are full of vitamins and nutrients that will leave your body feeling great. You'll have energy, which will allow you to stay active (it is also important that you remain active, as this will also help reset your body). Being active will help with your heart health, keep your metabolism working properly, and even help with digestion. It will be much easier to be active on the alkaline diet, as you will be consuming foods that will properly fuel you, as opposed to eating junk that will simply give you short-term energy (and cause you to crash later).

When resetting your body, it is important that you aren't dramatic with your diet. It is wise to slowly transition into it, as your body needs to adjust. If you live on junk right now, it may be difficult to dive into a plant-based diet. Your body will have developed a dependency on fried and sweetened foods, so that will be its primary source of energy. It will have been trained to extract its energy from such foods and will need to adjust to the new diet and reset itself. At first, you may feel tired. This may last for the first few weeks, as your body is resetting and adjusting to this new source of energy. Once you have adjusted, though, you will start to feel amazing and livelier again.

You must make sure that you are getting enough energy at all times. Fruits and vegetables are less densely concentrated in calories, so you will have to eat more of them to be equal to the number of calories you were receiving. If you were above your optimal caloric intake, which is common to many that aren't on a plant-based diet, you will need to adjust to how much food you should be eating. Be sure to consult a doctor, as they can take your lifestyle (and other factors such as weight, height, age, etc.) into consideration when figuring out what the best amount of food is for you. If you have been consuming more than you should, it will certainly take time for your body to reset and get used to this new way of life.

When resetting, it is important that you stay hydrated. You may want to consult your doctor to figure out how much water your body needs daily, but typically 8 eight-ounce glasses of water are what is recommended. This will vary based on your weight, height, age, activity level, and other factors. However, this is a good number to aim for, as most people are dehydrated. It is important to stay hydrated during the reset phase because your body will need all of the energy it can to be able to take care of you the best that it can. Drinking water also works to wash out any toxins that are in your body at the present.

For the alkaline diet, you will need to cut out the coffee. Many people, whether they know it or not, become addicted to it once they start regularly consuming it. Your body becomes dependent on it and is unable to function properly without it. Coffee is acid-producing and is not healthy. Although there are health benefits in coffee beans, the caffeine in coffee can lead to headaches, lost sleep, and an energy imbalance. Your body will need to adjust to being without coffee, and you may experience the side effects of being off of coffee. You may get headaches, lethargy, and energy spikes. This is normal and will have to be overcome to reset your body.

Resetting your body is a lengthy and gradual process. It will take a few weeks and may be difficult at first. However, it is necessary for your body to adjust to better foods and will be beneficial for your health.

Rebalance

You will also have to rebalance your body, which can be achieved via the alkaline diet. This will take time as well. Your body's pH will be unbalanced with the mass consumption of acid-producing foods. When switching to alkaline-promoting foods, your body will experience a rebalance. You will feel much better after this. Your body will be healed from the unbalanced, acidic state that it was in. It will help your entire body. You will be able to digest your food properly and will experience less indigestion, nausea, and bloating. You will have better heart health, and your blood will be healthier. Your immune system will be stronger, allowing your body to better defend you against sickness. Your respiratory system will be balanced, which will let you breathe better; your lungs will also be healthier.

Your muscular system will be stronger, allowing you to perform better and stay active. Activities won't be as strenuous anymore, and you will be able to move with ease. Your skeletal system will be healthier, and your risk for arthritis will be decreased. This will make the move easy and painless for you.

Your skin, hair, and nails will be healthier. Your skin will be clearer, your hair will be less oily, and your nails will be visibly healthier. This is because your skin will be getting the right foods that will make it look its best. Your nervous system will feel better and will help your physical, mental, and emotional health.

The new energy that you will have can really help your nervous system. Your excretory system will also thrive.

Your kidneys will be much healthier with the increase in water. Your body will be less acidic, allowing it to function properly. Your reproductive health will be better, and the chance of infertility and birth defects will be decreased. Overall, your health will be much better.

With rebalancing, there is more than just the physical aspect of it. You must also be mentally rebalanced. You must develop a balance between work and leisure. Make sure that you take time for yourself to enjoy yourself. This will help decrease your stress. If you are stressed, then your diet won't be able to fix your health. The health detriments caused by stress can cause serious consequences. Your diet will allow you to do this, though. Instead of feeling exhausted and having no energy, you will be able to enjoy your free time instead of spending it all sleeping and trying to regain energy. The nutrients that you will receive from the alkaline diet will allow you to rebalance your time.

In rebalancing your body, the alkaline diet is amazing. Your pH will be reset, as will the nutrients in your body. Instead of being deficient and therefore unbalanced in certain vitamins and minerals, your body will be balanced and be much healthier. This is the second stage in the "reset, rebalance, reconnect" system that is established by the alkaline diet. While your body resets, it is getting rid of any junk and its leftovers. This means that you are ready for rebalancing, in which you are transitioning from junk to alkaline foods. This will prepare you for reconnecting with the proper foods. As your body is rebalancing, it is transitioning. This is the state where your body will change. It may be difficult for you, as your body had previously been adjusted to the junk that it had. It had adjusted to its unbalanced state. By bringing your body back to a balanced state, you are optimizing your health. Your body systems will be able to work together better and make you the healthiest that you can possibly be.

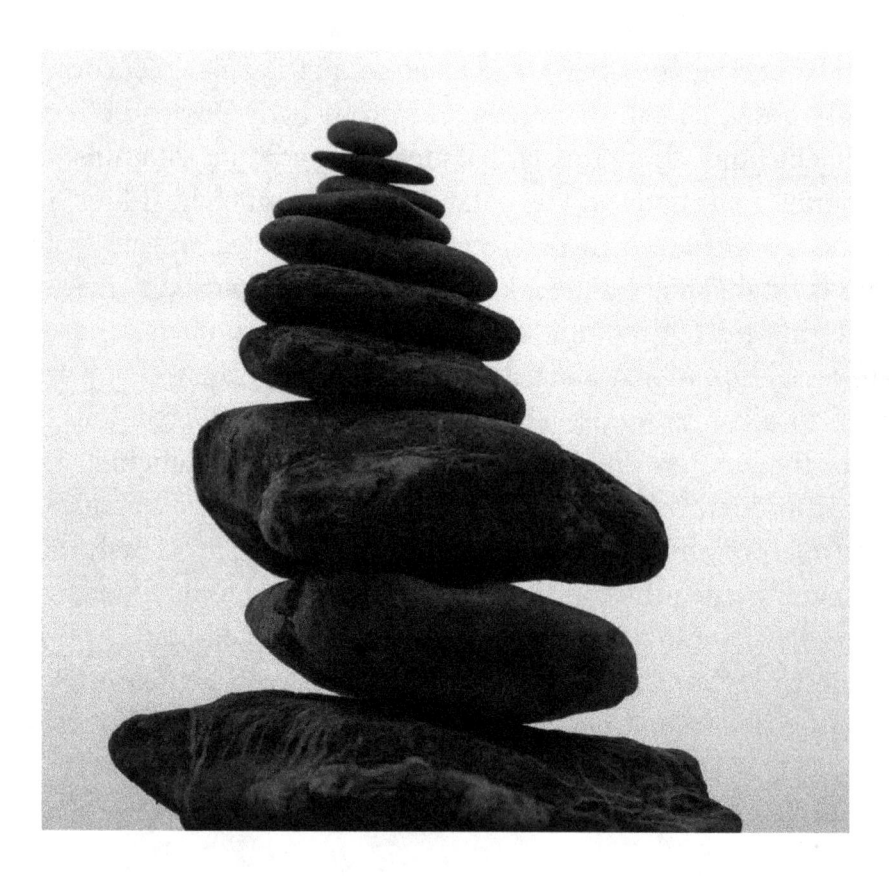

When getting rebalanced, you will experience some negative side effects that are left over from when your body was unbalanced. This is normal, and the transitional phase between resetting and reconnecting lasts at least a few weeks. But once you are transitioned to a healthy diet, you will no longer feel as tired, bloated, and stressed. You may also lose weight during this time. Your skin may break out a bit at first while your body is adjusting. But after, your skin will glow and be clearer than it's ever been.

Reconnect

These days, it seems like the only thing that we're connected to is the Internet. We spend so much time on our devices that we barely connect with the outside world. Overwhelmed with advertisements and bad influences, we are stuck in a world of junk and junk food. It is important to reconnect with the world around you. You must get into the new diet and connect your body with the right foods. Once you have gotten accustomed to the proper diet, your body will be reconnected. This is the third phase in the "reset, rebalance, and reconnect" transition from junk to health. By reconnecting with the foods that your body is made to consume, you are ensuring that you are the healthiest that you can possibly be. You will feel right because you are connected with the foods that you are supposed to be getting.

Perhaps you have slipped into bad habits. You have become inactive, have stopped watching what you eat, and are overwhelmed with stress. When stressed, we tend to forget to take care of ourselves, which leads to further stress. When you do this, you become detached from your body. You aren't paying attention to what your body needs, and you aren't taking care of it properly. With the alkaline diet, you become more aware of your body, how it operates, and what it needs. This allows you to become reconnected with your body. You will become more aware of it. When you are connected with your body, you will know when something isn't right. It won't be normal for you to not feel good! You will feel good about your body. Your self-confidence will go up. Because you are aware of what you are putting into your body and making sure that it is purely good stuff going into your body, you will be able to feel good about your body. You will be able to fuel your body properly and have enough energy to do everything that you want to do. You won't feel bad about your body anymore. This will help you mentally. The reconnecting phase is all about recovering from the pre-reset body that you had and about switching your mentality to being able to be "connected" with your body. You won't just eat for fun; you'll eat to make your body feel good and fueled with the proper foods. You will know exactly what's going on instead of remaining ignorant of the state in which your body is in. You will be able to figure out what you want to do.

With reconnecting, it is also important to figure out what changes you would like to make to your body. With a better diet, the possibilities are endless! You can now accomplish anything that you want! Whatever your way of reconnecting with your body is, make sure that you go with that. It will help you to stick to your diet more if you have a routine and ensure that you do what makes you happy. Do what makes you feel yourself. If dressing well makes you feel good about yourself and allows you to express yourself, do that. Some people prefer peace that meditation and yoga offer them. Some find that journaling helps them to write down all of their emotions and feel saner. Finding some sort of hobby for yourself will allow you to reconnect with your best self. If your diet has slipped, then it is likely that other aspects of your health, physical and mental, have slipped as well. That is why it is so important to reconnect with yourself and think about what it is that truly makes you happy. This will help you to be your best self. If you are your best self, you will be able to feel healthy and accomplish all of the goals that you set for yourself. If you feel good, you will be more determined and happier. Every day will be a positive experience for you, as opposed to a struggle.

The alkaline diet can help you to reconnect with your body. When you get your diet together, other aspects of your life will all come to order. You will be more at peace with the way you are, and you will feel good about yourself. These feelings will carry over to other aspects of your life and allow you to feel good about yourself. Instead of simply inhabiting your body, you will be able to live in it to its full potential. You will be in control of your body, as opposed to your body taking control of you.

While you are resetting your diet, it is wise to reset other aspects of your body. This will help you to maximize the benefits of reconnecting. You will be more aware of what you want instead of feeling disconnected from the world and your own thoughts. In this age of productivity and technology, self-care is more important than ever. You must make sure that you are taking care of your physical and mental health. You can't become disconnected from your body and let it control you.

One way to reconnect with your thoughts and the world is to reduce screen time. These days, it is very easy to keep scrolling on social media and keep clicking on fun ways to pass the time. Although there are many beneficial opportunities that technology offers us (such as reading and learning), there are also many unnecessary things out there that only serve as a waste of time. By managing your time wisely and only spending it on what matters to you, you are helping your mental health. You must also listen to your body. If you need rest, then it is important to rest. If you are dehydrated, drink water (although you should drink enough water to where you never reach the point of dehydration). Another way to reconnect is to get outdoors and be active.

This will allow you to get out into the real world and enjoy your surroundings. Additionally, it helps to take "pure" time to yourself. This means taking some time to just think and not have any distractions around you. Perhaps you can do this while taking a walk or getting outdoors. However, you must ensure that you have time without any other distractions, even music or technology of any sort. This will allow your thoughts to be clear and let you realize what it is that you truly want in life without your thoughts being scattered about. When you reconnect with your body, you will feel much better both physically and mentally.

How the Body Defends Itself

The immune system is the body's way of defending itself. Anything that passes through the skin must face the immune system. Anything that attacks our bodies (bacteria, viruses, parasites, and other microbes) must defend itself against our immune system. This system is spread out throughout our entire body, and it never stops working. It identifies which cells are ours and which are outsiders that must be attacked. These cells are eliminated, as they are a threat to the body. White blood cells, also known as leukocytes, circulate in the blood and are the ones who are on the hunt for potentially harmful cells. If they spot an enemy, they will multiply and signal others in the blood to follow. There are several places where white blood cells are stored. These areas are known as lymphoid organs and include the thymus, spleen, bone marrow, and lymph nodes. There are two types of white blood cells: phagocytes and lymphocytes.

Phagocytes attack pathogens and break them down. Lymphocytes recognize if cells are enemies or not based on the history of pathogens in the body.

When the immune system is working properly, it can prevent infections and illnesses. There are three types of immunity. There is innate immunity, which is what you are born with. This means that the types of illnesses and infections that you are subject to are typically human-specific, and your body is naturally defended from sicknesses that occur in other animals. This also includes how your skin and mucous naturally filter out potential threats from entering your body in the first place. The second type of immunity is called adaptive immunity. This is constantly developing. The lymphocytes build their knowledge of what is and aren't an enemy, and they building knowledge of how to defeat the different types of enemies. Throughout time, your body builds its immunity and is able to defend itself against more potential threats. The third type of immunity is passive immunity. This immunity is only temporary, and it is borrowed from a source (such as how a mother's milk will grant their baby immunity from diseases that the mother is immune to).

There can be problems with the immune system. Immunodeficiency disorders arise when there is some sort of deficiency within the immune system. This can occur from birth. It may also be acquired through infection or the use of drugs. Secondary immunodeficiency can occur from an improper diet, disease, or other problems with the body. Autoimmune disorders occur when the immune system starts attacking itself. This is the result of one of the body's own cells being identified as a harmful outsider. Allergies occur when the immune system overreacts to certain substances. Substances that are harmless to others will cause the immune system to overreact and cause symptoms to arise. The fourth main problem with the immune system is cancer. This occurs when cells grow beyond the scope that they are supposed to. These problems can all be dangerous for the body and cause a variety of problems and symptoms to arise.

When the immune system is healthy, it will be able to properly execute the immune response. The immune response is the entire method of defense that the immune system uses to rid itself of potentially harmful objects and cells. It begins by detecting which cells are and are not welcome in the body. Once an antigen (a cell that is recognized as unwelcome by lymphocytes) is seen, lymphocytes secrete antibodies, which will attach themselves to antigens. This "marks" the cell. Once the cell is marked, it is attacked and destroyed. A healthy immune system will be able to properly identify which cells are harmful, and they will be able to successfully get rid of them. The immune system is amazing, and it is very powerful and effective at what it does.

With the alkaline diet, your body will be able to reset, rebalance, and reconnect. You will also be able to defend yourself from sickness, as your immune system will work properly. By starting the alkaline diet, you are ensuring that your body is working properly, and it is able to be the healthiest that it can be. That includes resetting itself from any junk that it was consuming, rebalancing its pH and nutrients in it, and reconnecting itself to you. You will also be able to defend yourself against illness and infections effectively. With the alkaline diet, your body will be healthy.

Chapter 5

Acid-Forming Foods and Habits to Avoid

With the alkaline diet, there are certain foods that you should try to avoid. These foods are acid-forming and will leave your body unbalanced. Acidic foods contribute to a variety of health problems. There are also habits that you should avoid. Avoiding these habits will help you to be healthier overall and will help your body to operate optimally.

Foods to Avoid

There are certain foods that you should avoid. Otherwise, you are not following the alkaline diet and ensuring maximum health. These foods are acidic and will cause more acidity in your body. These foods have a pH level of 4.6 or below. One type of food that you should limit is anything with grains. This includes any bread or such. These foods are not only acid-producing foods but are also loaded with carbohydrates. They should be limited as much as possible for maximum health.

Foods with added sugar and sodium should also be avoided. Sugar is added in almost every food there is! That is, for processed foods. The obvious foods that are sugary to avoid are sweets such as cookies, cakes, and doughnuts. However, they are added in almost everything. Even though applesauce may seem healthy, it typically contains a large amount of added sugar. It's much better to just eat the real thing! If you aren't eating the natural fruit or vegetable, you are most likely eating food with unnecessary added sugar (or sodium). This sugar leads to acidity in the body, and it is converted to fat. It's just better to avoid added sugar. Foods with high added sodium lead to hypertension or high blood pressure. This is not good for you, and these foods should be avoided as much as possible.

Dairy products are best to be avoided. Even though dairy is typical in many people's diets, it shouldn't be. Milk in mammals is made for the offspring of that animal. Breast milk in humans is made for human babies to drink as they grow and develop. Cow milk is made for calves. However, humans started consuming cow milk and haven't stopped coming up with new ways to incorporate it into their diets! It is unnatural for us to drink cow milk. Furthermore, many people are lactose intolerant (unable to digest cow milk properly). This means that your body can't properly consume it without feeling unwell. Although most people have it so slight that they barely even notice, it is found in most people. It is especially found in those with Asian backgrounds. Europeans have been found to have the greatest resistance to it. Even if you are only slightly allergic to it, consuming cow milk is not worth the risks.

It is best to avoid meat and fish as much as possible. These foods, even when fresh and sourced properly, are acid-producing. These days, meat is typically sourced improperly. The conditions for raising animals are terrible, as many animals are shoved into small spaces. Disease easily spreads this way. Additionally, the animals have many hormones added to them to enhance and speed up their growth. They are also typically bred at a young age (too young to be healthy and fully sexually mature). This is not the food that you want to put in your body.

Processed foods and fast foods should be avoided. These foods are mass-produced and typically contain many elements of the other foods that should be avoided. Anything that is in a package and doesn't contain the pure food that it is from should be avoided. Any "snack" food such as chips, pretzels, or crackers should not be consumed. These specific foods are loaded with carbohydrates and added sodium. They are also acid-producing. Fast foods should be avoided. They only rarely offer options that are good for your health. Typically, these foods are served at restaurants and include food such as fried chicken, French fries, and cheeseburgers. There are also fast, frozen meals. These are loaded with preservatives, sodium, and sugar. They are almost never whole foods.

Beverages besides water should be avoided. If everyone were to drink water and water only, obesity could be greatly reduced. Unnecessary sugar in the body is converted to fat. Sodas have been found to lead to a great variety of health problems. The carbonation leads to extra gas in the body, and the syrup found in colas and other sodas has been found to lead to cancer. Beverages such as lemonade, tea, and juice have an incredible amount of added sugar in them. Sweetened tea has also been linked to the development of kidney stones. Energy drinks are not good for your body and have even been linked to the occurrence of heart attacks. Drinks containing caffeine are not healthy for your sleep and lead to spikes and drops of energy.

Alcohol is also acid-producing and should be avoided. Water is the best drink to consume.

It is important to avoid adding supplements, sweeteners, and salt to your food unnecessarily. Foods that contain extremely high levels of protein in them should also be avoided. Most often, the consumption of these foods leads to an over-indulgence of protein. The surplus of a macronutrient is unhealthy. Additionally, these are acid-producing foods. It is also best to avoid extra sweeteners and salts. The mixes that you flavor your water with, table salt that you add to your food, and other such ingredients should be avoided to ensure a healthier body.

Habits to Avoid

Even if you are consuming all of the right foods, you still need to establish proper eating habits. Otherwise, you aren't maximizing your health the proper way and may not be experiencing all of the benefits that healthy eating offers. By ensuring that you have a proper eating schedule and are following certain eating rules, you will be able to feel better and be healthier.

- First and most importantly, be sure to start every day with a good breakfast. It is said that breakfast is the most important meal of the day, and it's true. After an extended period of sleeping, you must start out with a meal to kick your metabolism into action. You must make sure that it is a nutritious and filling meal, and that you accompany it with a glass or two of water. This will start your day off well and ensure that you are establishing good habits from the moment you wake up.

- Also, you must ensure that you are waking up from receiving a proper amount of sleep. When you rest, your body takes time to repair and recover. Your body gains back its energy, does any tasks that it needs to do, and leaves you feeling refreshed. You must ensure that you get the proper amount of sleep because too much or too little can prove very harmful for your health. It is typically recommended that you receive eight hours of sleep at night, but that will depend on your age. At a very young age, children and babies are recommended to get a higher amount of sleep. As you age, six to seven hours is optimal, rising again to seven to eight with even more age. The proper amount of sleep will allow your body to digest its food properly and keep your metabolism performing at its best. Fatigue can also lead to overeating, so it is best to avoid that.
- Make sure that you eat your meals while seated and free of distractions. Consuming foods while standing up, laying down, or while in motion can lead to improper digestion. You should also eat your food without any distractions. Otherwise, you can overeat and not be aware of what you are putting into your body. You will also be hungrier later, as you will not realize how much food you have eaten.
- Ensure that you don't overeat. If you are full, stop eating. It is okay to not finish the food you make; you can always finish it later.
- Drink enough water. Often, you only think you are hungry because you are dehydrated and need water. Drinking water will keep you full for longer, and your body will be able to properly work and digest food.

- Stop having such large portions. It helps to start eating on smaller plates. That way, you can limit yourself and feel like you're eating more when you're actually eating the same amount.
- It is okay to snack. It is usually recommended to eat a few small meals every few hours instead of two or three large meals spread throughout the day. This will keep your energy up, and you won't ever reach the point where you feel the need to over consume or binge.
- Try flavoring your food with herbs and spices instead of condiments and sauces.
- Give yourself a cut-off time for eating. You shouldn't consume any food within an hour of going to sleep.
- Don't eat junk food when experiencing negative emotions. Instead, substitute it for a healthy snack (such as fruit). Or, find a better way to deal with your troubles. Talk to a friend, go for a walk, listen to music, or take a bath. Eating junk will further perpetuate the problem and make you feel even worse.
- Don't eat too quickly. Your brain will not have time to register everything that you are putting in your body, and you may not realize that you are full. Take small bites and eat slowly.

Consequences of an Acid-Alkaline Imbalance

It is necessary for your body to have the proper acid-alkaline balance in order to function at its fullest potential. The kidneys and lungs are the primary ones keeping this in check, and they must be taken care of properly to ensure that you are healthy. If it is not maintained, even if it is slightly off, your organs won't be able to function the way that they should. Your blood will not be healthy, which can lead to heart problems. Your lungs can develop respiratory acidosis, which can lead to confusion, lethargy, and difficulty breathing. You may also develop metabolic acidosis, which is where your kidneys may not remove the excess of acid in your body due to its great surplus. If left untreated, these issues can lead to serious health problems and even death. This is why it is crucial to watch your health and ensure that your acid and alkaline levels are properly balanced.

Each system in your body is affected by the acid-alkaline levels. Your digestive system must properly digest food, which can't be too acidic (or else your body won't be able to properly digest it). Your muscles and bones must be able to move properly and be strong, which can be inhibited by poor nutrition and high acid levels. Your circulatory system must be able to pump blood to your body without a problem, which can be determined by your acid-alkaline levels; if you have too much acid, then there can be problems with circulation. Your skin, the largest organ that your body has, is directly affected by what you eat. Your hair, teeth, nails, and skin are all direct reflections of your health. If you have too much acid, your appearance will reflect that.

It is crucial to make sure that your body does not have an acid-alkaline imbalance. If it does, a great number of health issues can arise. With the alkaline diet, you are ensuring that your body is functioning the proper way. It is important to avoid highly acidic foods and unhealthy habits to guarantee the best health for yourself possible.

Chapter 6

Benefits of the Alkaline Diet

It's no secret; eating a healthy diet will help you to have a healthier body. You'll feel better physically, mentally, and emotionally. It is extremely important to take care of your health. You will feel much better and be able to perform your everyday tasks with ease.

Physical Benefits

You will feel much better physically. If you were previously tired all the time and had no energy to perform everyday activities, you will not feel like that anymore. Instead of struggling to breathe every time you walk, you will be able to do whatever life throws at you. You will find it easier to stay active. Because of this, you will have a healthier body than you ever had before. You may lose weight. Your muscles will be stronger and recover more easily than before. Your bones will also be stronger and will be more able to combat the effects of aging, which will slow (or even stop) osteoarthritis from occurring. Your chance of osteoporosis will also be decreased. This means that you will be able to be active even after aging. You will also have a quicker recovery time. This will allow you to stay active every day and not get overly tired whenever you exercise.

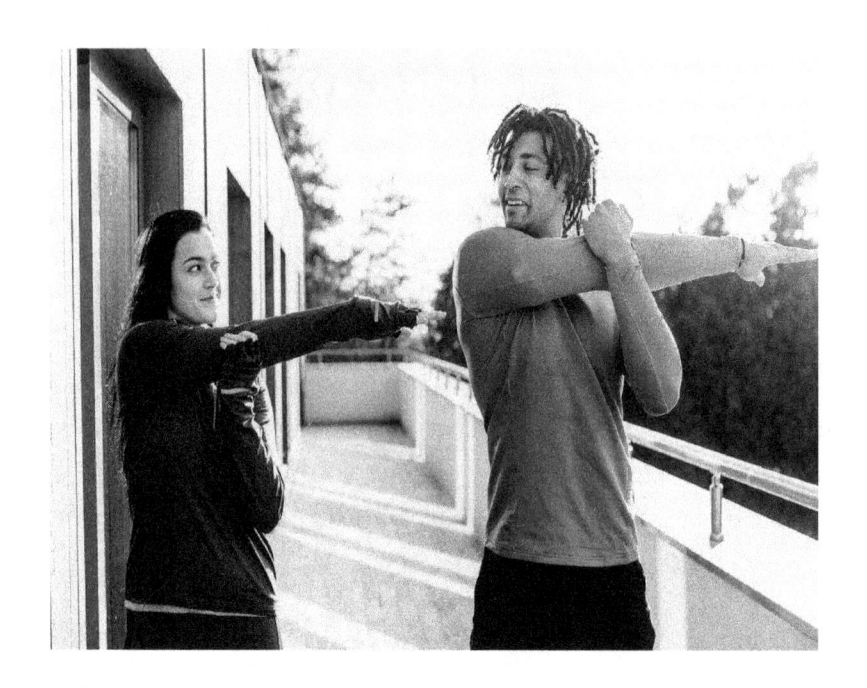

You will also look better physically. Your skin will be brighter, you will have less acne, and your skin may even glow. It will be less oily. Your hair will be shinier and not as greasy. Your nails will look healthier than ever. Your teeth will also be healthier. They will be stronger and will be less prone to rotting or developing other issues. Your body will be in better shape because you will be able to be active and will be able to be more active every day. Because of this, you may lose unnecessary weight. It will make your body look healthier.

Your body will also undergo its processes more efficiently and effectively. Your kidneys will be healthier due to the increase in water and decrease in acid-producing foods. It will be drastically different if you used to consume sugary, carbonated, caffeinated, or alcoholic beverages. The increased pH in your urine will help you to go to the bathroom effectively. This may also prevent issues from arising such as kidney stones and the like. The alkaline diet is also found to contribute to a reduced risk of cancer. It may also help you to be treated more easily from cancer. Cancer results from cells multiplying at an uncontrollable rate. This may occur from a weakened immune system; however, the alkaline diet helps to strengthen the immune system. It will help your white blood cells to more easily identify the difference between harmful and harmless cells, and it can help them to attack the cells that are harmful more effectively.

The alkaline diet will also help your heart health. If your blood is healthier, it will be able to circulate more easily. Your risk for high blood pressure will also be reduced. The alkaline diet further helps with pain.

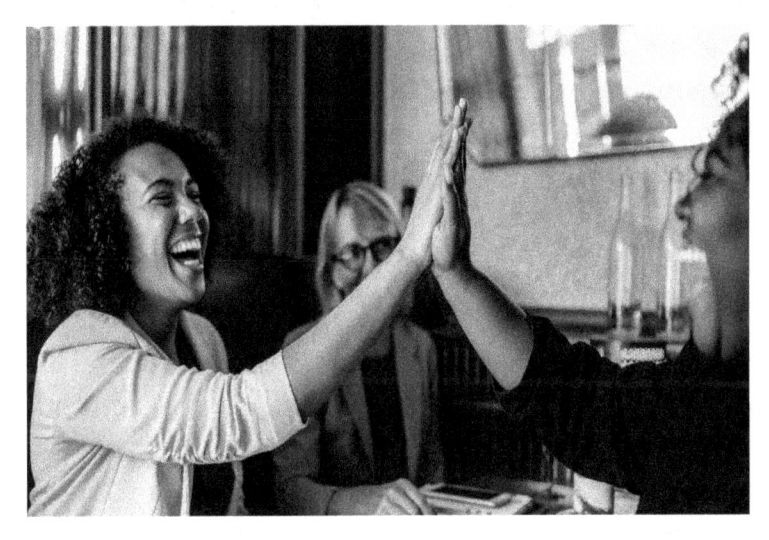

While eating junk food, your body is not receiving the proper nutrients required for repairing the body properly. When you eat the right foods, your body will be able to fix itself easily, and your pain will be reduced. Your digestive system will also be improved. You will be able to eat without worrying about any stomach or other digestive problems. Your food will be digested properly, and your body will thank you for it. Your metabolism will also be healthier, and you will be able to properly break down the food that you consume.

Your chances for developing certain diseases and other health problems will also be reduced. You will be less likely to have a stroke. You won't be as likely to have a heart attack. Your body will be receiving all of the proper things that it needs, and it won't be consuming the junk that will just bring it down. You won't have to worry about a long list of problems that you may develop.

Overall, your physical health will be much better with the alkaline diet. You will be able to enjoy life as it is without being worried about developing issues. Your body will work the way that it is supposed to. It is extremely important for you to take care of your body. If you do so, you will feel much better and will enjoy all of the benefits that eating healthy offers.

__Mental Benefits__

When eating a diet that's healthier, your mental health will be improved. You will be less likely to experience mental illnesses such as anxiety and depression. You will be able to think more clearly and will be less confused. Eating healthier foods will allow you to think very clearly. First off, you will experience the physical benefits of eating healthy. With the greater amount of energy that you have, you won't feel as moody anymore. When you aren't as tired, you will be able to think clearly and not have any health problems weighing you down. You will be able to concentrate better, as opposed to being distracted by exhaustion or having to deal with symptoms of physical health issues. When you eat junk food, your body is using its energy to trying to break down these foods and attempting to extract energy from these foods. However, these foods don't provide you with the nutrients and energy that you need to function properly. When you follow the alkaline diet, you won't have these issues.

Your brain is a part of your body. You must also take care of it. It is always thinking and needs the energy to function properly. When you fuel it the right way, your brain will operate optimally. As opposed to damaging your brain with junk, you will be feeding it what it needs to think well. Diets high in added sugars have been found to lead to impaired brain function.

Emotional Benefits

In addition to being able to think better, you will be emotionally better. Because you will have better physical and mental health, you will feel better emotionally. You will feel more emotionally stable. Previously, you may have felt guilty about the foods you consumed or felt self-conscious of your body. Once you start the alkaline diet, you will feel better because you will know exactly what you are putting into your body; they will all be good foods.

Your mood will be enhanced. This will allow you to have more energy, motivation, productivity, and creativity. The nutrients that you will be receiving more of will allow your brain to release more endorphins, making you happier. Deficiencies of nutrients lead to tiredness and depression. You will no longer have to worry about these issues; you will be a happier person.

You will also have more energy, which can directly lift your mood. You will feel more motivated to accomplish tasks, which will allow you to be more productive. This will lead to a greater sense of accomplishment, which will make you feel much better about yourself. You will also now have enough energy to do the things that may not have been possible before. For instance, you will be able to be more active. Being active and regularly exercising have been linked to being more emotionally well. You will also not experience crashes that overconsumption of sugar and caffeine may have caused you before. This will lead to greater consistency in your energy levels, which will help you to be more mentally well.

You will be able to learn more easily. Your increased mental health will allow you to concentrate better and help you to absorb information more easily. This will further lead to greater motivation and a higher sense of self-accomplishment. You will feel much better about yourself, as you will be able to accomplish many things that you were previously unable to. You will be able to learn more, go to more places, and meet more people. You may have had trouble talking to people before, and you may have even isolated yourself from people. This is common when you have low energy, self-esteem, and overall health. You will be able to build better and stronger relationships with people, which will greatly help your mood to be up and your mental health to be much greater. You will be yourself again.

Your serotonin levels will be more balanced. This neurotransmitter helps you to sleep well, have a proper appetite, have more stable moods, and fight pain more easily. Serotonin is primarily produced in the gastrointestinal tract. When you eat properly, your gastrointestinal health will be greater, which will allow your serotonin levels to be better regulated.

You will also be less stressed. You won't have to worry about eating properly, as all of the foods in your body will be good for you. Your risk for a variety of health problems will be greatly reduced, which can also lower your stress.

You will feel much better and will be able to concentrate on what matters in life. You won't find yourself in the constant cycle of eating, feeling better and energized temporarily, then crashing, and then eating again. You will be filling your body with the fuel that it needs to operate well from the start.

When people switch from eating junk to eating good foods, the change is almost instantaneous. You will immediately feel better. At first, it may be difficult, but it will be worth it. You will be so proud of having self-control and sticking to a diet. You will feel good about yourself and what you're putting into your body, and the food you consume will make you feel good, too.

Importance of Health

Every day, the choices on what you eat affect you. Not only will you feel better in the moment and have more energy, better mental health, and improved moods, but you are making choices that affect your entire life. You will be able to sleep better every night, which will lead to more energy every day and greater productivity as well. You will be able to accomplish more in a lesser amount of time. You will have a reduced risk of health problems. These problems could have lasting effects or even affect you for life. You will also live longer. With a decreased risk of health issues and an increased amount of energy and nutrients that help you to thrive, you will live a life that will be healthier and longer.

With a better diet, you will also be able to be more active. Instead of being unable to walk at a young age, you will be able to live the life you want for decades and decades. If you eat and exercise properly, you will be able to maintain a healthy weight. This will greatly reduce your risk for a number of health problems, as obesity can cause anything from bone issues to heart disease. You will certainly enjoy life much more.

Overall, your health is extremely important. You are only given one body, so you must treat it well. Your body requires fuel, and you must be able to fuel it with the right foods. If you don't, you are putting yourself at risk for a variety of problems. If you treat your body well, it will treat you well and you will be able to do what you would like, as opposed to being slowed down by everyday tasks.

The alkaline diet provides you with the proper diet to ensure maximum health. You will experience physical benefits. Your body will function better, you will look healthier, and your risk for health issues will be greatly decreased. You will also have better mental health. You will be able to concentrate, learn better, and think properly. Your emotional health will be better.

You will be more mentally stable, not experience awful moods as frequently, and will be happier overall. It is important to take care of your body and to stay healthy so that you can live the longest and healthiest life possible.

Chapter 7

Alkaline Foods to Enjoy

Most people tend to avoid diets because they fear that there won't be any foods for them to eat. They are also hesitant because they don't think that the foods that comply with the diet will be as tasty. This is clearly wrong, as the alkaline diet offers many options for foods to eat. It may be difficult to switch at first, as your body most likely isn't used to consuming a large amount of these regularly. However, you will eventually get used to it and learn to love these foods.

Alkaline Fruits

There are a large number of fruits that can be consumed while on the alkaline diet. These fruits are all alkaline-promoting. Even though some fruits (like lemons and oranges) are acidic, they promote alkalinity. This is important for your health. There is a large variety to choose from as far as fruits go.

There are high, medium, and low alkaline fruits. All of these are better for your health than most junk, but the high-alkaline fruits are the very best. These include blackberries, strawberries, raspberries, tangerines, nectarines, limes, papaya, pineapple, melons (watermelon, cantaloupe, and honeydew), mango, and passion fruit. All of these fruits are extremely delicious and can be easily incorporated into your diet.

The medium alkaline fruits include grapes, dried fruit (such as raisins, dates, etc.), oranges, blueberries, apples, apricots, avocado, bananas, green olives, pears, peaches, lemons, grapefruit, and cherries.

Coconuts have a low alkaline. However, all of these fruits are healthy. Fruits are able to provide you with the nutrients that you need to stay energized. It is recommended that you consume about two cups or more of fruit per day to keep you healthy. The fruit is not densely packed with calories, fat, or sodium. It is also a good way to get natural sugars. They are loaded with vitamins and nutrients such as fiber, vitamin C, folic acid, and potassium. Consuming fruit reduces your risk for heart attacks and strokes. They also reduce the chances of type-2 diabetes and obesity. You will also have lower blood pressure, a lesser risk of developing kidney stones, and decreased bone loss.

Because fruits aren't as densely packed in calories and fat as other foods (such as cheeseburgers) are, you can eat more of them and get the same number of calories and fat. If you enjoy eating a lot, this is highly beneficial for you. You won't have to worry about overeating and causing health problems for yourself.

Fruits are also delicious. They are typically sweet and make great additions to many dishes and such. You can infuse your water with fruit to add flavor to it. This is commonly done with lemons but is also popular with limes, strawberries, and oranges. It also looks nice! Certain juices are also good to consume, although you must ensure that it is pure juice. If there are any chemicals or sugars added, then it ruins the whole point of the juice. Fruit salads are also delicious. A bowl of grapes, melon, apples, strawberries, and oranges taste delicious together. You can throw all of your favorite fruit into a bowl and call it a day! It's super easy to make, and you don't have to worry about cooking or preparing the food any special way. Dried fruit makes for a delicious snack. You can even make a "trail mix" with dried peaches, dried pineapples, and raisins. This is delicious and will keep you filled and fueled. A bowl of fruit is also yummy. Chopped bananas, watermelon cubes, and orange slices are a few of the snack options that are delicious. Watermelon slices are also amazing for hot summer days, as they have high water content and will keep you hydrated.

Make sure that you incorporate a variety of fruits into your diet. It is commonly said that you should keep your plate colorful. This is because foods with certain pigments have specific health benefits. Red, purple, and blue fruits are great antioxidants. They help your heart and brain to operate well. Orange and yellow fruits help to maintain eye health, fight cancer, and keep your skin healthy. White fruits (such as bananas); provide you with vitamin C, folic acid, and fiber.

The consumption of fruits is very important for your diet. It is also important to ensure that you are eating a variety of fruits so that you can stay healthy and balanced. Overall, though, the fruit is amazing for your health.

Alkaline Veggies

There are also a number of vegetables that can be consumed while on the alkaline diet. Just like with fruit, there are high, medium, and low-alkaline vegetables. All vegetables are going to be loaded with nutrients and lead to better health, however. It is recommended that you consume around three cups of vegetables per day. This will help the acidity in your body to be balanced. Vegetables are packed with vitamins and minerals that will help you to have the best health that you can.

Vegetables with high alkaline include celery, onions, asparagus, collard greens, parsnips, kale, and sweet potatoes. These vegetables are amazing for you and will help to balance your pH well.

Vegetables with a medium alkaline include artichokes, beets, baked potatoes, bell peppers, broccoli, eggplant, summer squash, zucchini, okra, and cabbage.

Vegetables with a low alkaline include snow peas, carrots, cucumbers, mushrooms, cauliflower, and Brussels sprouts. Although these have a lower alkaline, they are still healthy and will provide you with the nutrients that you need to be healthy.

A diet full of vegetables is amazing for your health. They provide you with many vitamins and other nutrients such as potassium, fiber, folic acid, vitamin A, vitamin E, and vitamin C. When eating vegetables, you will experience better health and a reduction in the likelihood of health issues. You will have a decreased risk of high blood pressure. You will also have reduced cholesterol levels and a decreased risk of heart disease. Your risk for cancer, stroke, and type-2 diabetes will also be reduced.

It is also important to consume a variety of vegetables. The colors are the same as fruits, yet vegetables also have leafy greens. These contain vitamin A and potassium. Vegetables will help to eliminate bloat by flushing out the toxins in your body. Your digestive system will run more smoothly, and you won't experience constipation. Vegetables are also helpful for having clearer skin. The vitamin C and water contained in vegetables helps to reduce wrinkles and keep skin hydrated.

Once you start eating more vegetables, you may notice that your skin has a natural glow to it. That's a result from beta carotene. Vegetables will also help to decrease stress. The magnesium, vitamin B, and omega-3 fatty acids that are in vegetables also help to fight anxiety and depression. Veggies are helpful for ensuring healthier mental health. Vegetables will actually relax your blood, which will lower your blood pressure.

The fiber in vegetables will help you to maintain your blood sugar levels, which will keep your energy and mood balanced. Your bones will thank you for eating vegetables. Due to the calcium, vitamin D, vitamin K, magnesium, potassium, and prebiotic fiber, your bones will be healthier and stronger than ever once you start consuming vegetables. Your overall health will be greatly increased by the consumption of vegetables. You will look, think, and feel better. You will experience the benefits of healthy eating and the decreased risk of health problems.

It's quite easy to incorporate vegetables into your diet. Perhaps the most common method of eating veggies is by salads. This is a way that you can add in a bunch of vegetables and eat them all at once. You may even add additional ingredients for further flavor. You can also make smoothies from vegetables. Green smoothies are delicious and look appealing as well. They are a great way to eat many vegetables at once, especially if you don't have much time to eat. You may also make smoothie bowls, which are fun to make and delicious to eat. Soup is another way to incorporate your vegetables. You may throw in foods that typically wouldn't work well together and create a delicious soup. Soup is also refreshing for cool winter days. It is important to fit all of the vegetables you need into the day, so it is wise to consider choosing vegetables as snacks. Carrots and celery make amazing snack foods, especially when on the go. You can also turn vegetables into noodles. Zucchini is popular for this and can be a way to still enjoy pasta without the acidity. To enjoy sandwiches, you can opt for lettuce wraps instead of bread. You may also bake vegetables to turn them into chips.

Vegetables are very healthy for you. They provide you with a number of health benefits and prevent health issues from arising. Veggies are also delicious. There are many ways that you can enjoy them. Vegetables are delicious and healthy.

Other Alkaline Foods & Alkaline Water

There are other foods that are alkaline besides fruits and vegetables. Soy products are great to incorporate into your diet. Miso, soybeans, tofu, and tempeh are wonderful to eat and are healthy. Certain dairy is okay to have in your diet, as long as it is unsweetened (milk and yogurt). Dairy should be avoided overall, but it is okay to eat unsweetened milk and yogurt. You may also add herbs and spices to your food for additional flavor. Just make sure you aren't adding salt, mustard, or nutmeg. Any other herbs and spices are pretty much all good. Cilantro and oregano are great to add to vegetables and help them to taste great. You may also choose to add sea salt, ginger root, parsley, black pepper, basil, garlic, cinnamon, bay leaf, and cayenne pepper to your foods. Beans and lentils are good to add to your diet, and they offer a variety of different options for you to pair with your food. Although you should avoid most grains and bread, some whole grains are actually good to eat. Millet, quinoa, and amaranth are all good to eat. You may also opt for unsweetened granola, oatmeal, and wild rice. You can also add certain other things to your food such as olive oil, avocados, nuts, and seeds. You may cook your food in olive oil. Other oils, such as flax oil, coconut oil, avocado oil, and cod liver oil, can also be consumed. Nuts and seeds can be added to salads. You can add pumpkin seeds, chestnuts, cashews, almonds, sesame seeds, and sunflower seeds. There are many options for mixing and matching alkaline foods. You don't have to just eat fruits and vegetables. It's easy to add flavor, texture, and a greater variety to your meals.

There are also certain beverages besides water that you may consume and will still be alkaline. Herbal teas are perfect. They have also been shown to be calming and be good for your health. Ginger tea is great and has a high alkaline level. You may also opt for green tea. Mineral water is also good to drink. Certain juices, if they are unsweetened, can also be good to consume. Grapefruit and pineapple juices are okay to consume. Apple juice, grape juice, and orange juice are also alright to consume every so often. It is important that you mostly drink water, but it is possible to switch it up a bit.

As far as water goes, there are different types of water. Although most water tastes the same to the general population, there has been a recent trend of drinking alkaline water. This water has a higher pH than regular water. Most water has a pH level of about 6.5 to 7.5. Alkaline water has a higher pH than this. It has been claimed to help celebrities to maintain their health and is a fad diet essential. The business of alkaline water has multiplied by ten from 2014 to 2017. One of the highest brands, perhaps the highest, has water with a pH of about 9.5. Alkaline water is said to increase your body's pH, similarly to how the alkaline diet works. It has not been directly proven that alkaline water significantly helps your body's pH levels much more than regular water. Water is the perfect beverage to drink. However, alkaline water has a slightly higher pH than normal water. Every bit counts, right? It has not been proven that alkaline water causes significant differences from regular water, yet adding alkaline water might push your body just that little bit more. Coupled with the alkaline diet, your body will be healthy. Alkaline water certainly won't hurt. It contains alkalizing compounds such as calcium, silica, potassium, magnesium, and bicarbonate. These nutrients will help provide your body with the proper ingredients it needs to function to its fullest potential.

You will be preventing acidosis, which causes heart issues, hormonal fluctuations, and muscle/bone loss. Your body will have more nutrients and fewer toxins in it, which will help your body to function properly. There has been evidence suggesting that alkaline water is linked to an increase in overall body alkalinity. It is also helpful for your kidneys. You will have urine with a higher pH. You will also have a decreased risk for kidney stones and other issues with your kidneys.

It is important to vary the water you drink, though. Because alkaline water contains a good amount of minerals, you must be sure that you don't drink too much. Consuming too many of these minerals will lead to a buildup of them in your body, which can be harmful. So, you must have both regular water and alkaline water to ensure that your health is the greatest.

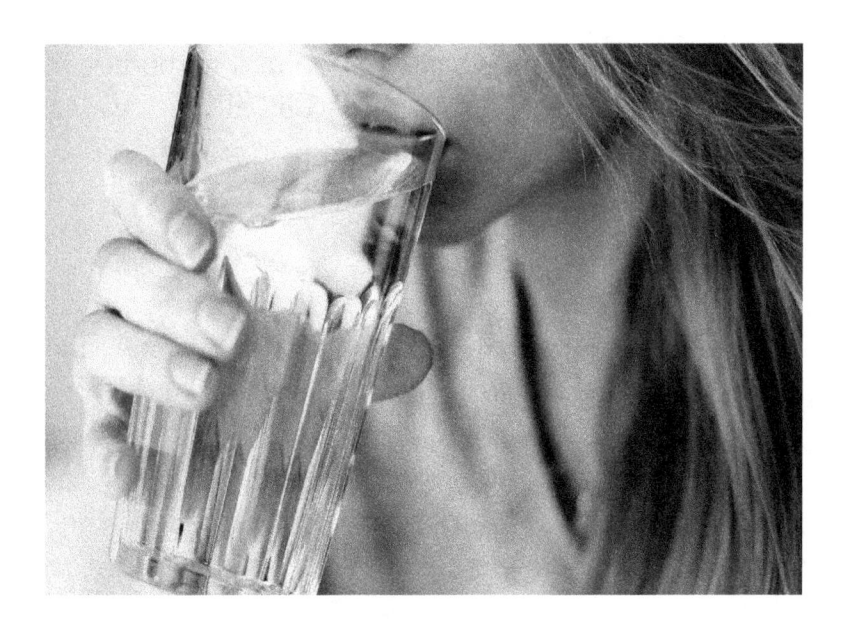

Alkaline water is helpful for athletes, though. When being active, you need extra nutrients to keep you going throughout your activities. It can help your circulatory system to more efficiently pump blood. You may also have decreased urine output and blood osmolality. You will be properly hydrated for any activities that you wish to do. Your muscles will thank you for the minerals that they are now receiving, and you may also have more energy. It will help you to not be as fatigued. More hydrogen ions are produced when you exercise, so drinking alkaline water can help your body to buffer properly and have a more balanced pH. It is especially helpful for long-term exercisers. This means that if you are a marathoner, alkaline water is great for you and will provide you with the energy that you need to stay active for long periods of time. Alkaline water also serves as a toxin preventer. It neutralizes toxins that may be found in regular water. When tap water is disinfected, some of the disinfectants mix with organic matter and form disinfectant by-products. These by-products can be broken down by alkaline water, keeping our bodies free of toxins. Your gut will also be disinfected by alkaline water, and you will be further protected from dangerous microbes. Your liver will also be healthier due to alkaline water's ability to lower glycation levels.

Alkaline water has also been shown to slow the aging process, cleanse the colon, support the immune system, and help the skin to be clearer. It has also been shown to detoxify and hydrate. It also prevents harmful health issues such as obesity and cancer. Alkaline water, coupled with the alkaline diet, can help you to be healthier. It makes sense to not only regulate the food that goes into your body but to also regulate the pH of the water that you drink. Hydration is important.

Alkaline Meals

There are many meals that you can make from alkaline-friendly foods. You don't have to just consume raw fruits and vegetables all day, every day. You can make fruit and veggie salads. Fruit salads are very yummy and are also usually very sweet. Vegetable salads are common, and you can enhance it. Adding sesame or sunflower seeds adds a crunch to the salad and will also enhance the flavor. You may also add fruit, such as orange slices, for an added sweetness. Salads are delicious and very easy to make. You can also make them ahead of time for a quick meal on the go.

Smoothie bowls have received a lot of attention lately. The recent trend is eating acai bowls. These are made from a smoothie blend of acai and typically contain granola, fruits, and seeds on top. These are great because they look appealing, which will encourage you to eat them. They are also fun to make and easy to customize. You can choose which fruit you would like to put on top and add as much or as little as you would like. You can also choose some seeds to add on top. You may even opt for different smoothie blends on the bottom, and you can opt for a fruit and veggie blend for added health benefits.

Pasta is a great choice. You can make pasta yourself from zucchini. You may also make your own sauce from vegetables, or even mix the pasta with olive oil if you want to add some more fat to the meal. Herbs and spices are necessities when it comes to pasta. Oregano, parsley, basil, rosemary, and cilantro all taste great. Garlic and onion do as well. You may add mushrooms and a dash of cinnamon, too. Broccoli also tastes good with pasta. This, again, is very easy to customize.

You may also make wraps. Lettuce wraps are delicious, especially with grilled mushrooms and spinach inside. Coupled with oregano, you have one very tasty meal.

There are many ways to mix and match the foods that you can eat while on the alkaline diet. The food is all delicious, and you aren't limited when it comes to food. Alkaline water is also worth a try. You might as well go all the way with putting alkaline goods into your body! It is very fun and tasty to eat in compliance with the alkaline diet.

Chapter 8

Troubleshooting

When starting a diet, you will face difficulties. It will be hard to start off and build the habit. It is often said that it takes about thirty days to build a habit, so the first few weeks will be rough. You will need to adjust to a new diet and you may experience some hardships during the first few weeks of the new diet. Your body must have time to adjust. You will also, especially at first, crave the junk that you used to eat. It will be hard to stay on your diet with holidays, social events, and the like. It is possible, though. You must also ensure that you are eating enough and getting enough of the nutrients that you need.

The First Few Weeks

The first few weeks of your diet will be rough. You will need time to adjust to a dietary change, as your body will have gotten used to the foods that you regularly put in your body. Many people switch what they eat without taking proper care of themselves. They go all into the diet, and they forget basic self-care. They end up starving themselves. People also don't speak to a medical professional beforehand and get an opinion on how to properly go about the diet. These mistakes lead to a hard time with the diet.

During the first few weeks of a new diet, your body will go through the adjustment period. You have developed a dependency on the foods that you used to consume and having new food into your diet while getting rid of the old food will shock your body. You are providing it with a new energy source.

You will most likely feel very tired and worn out. This is because your body is not used to extracting energy from these new sources. If you switch from a primarily fast-food, meat-based diet to a fresh, plant-based diet, your body will not know what to do at first. Perhaps you still occasionally ate plant-based foods, but your body will be especially shocked if you ate a diet rich in meat. This is because when you do have meals that are plant-based, your body will still be waiting for you to provide it with the meat that it uses for energy.

Perhaps you ate a lot of bread and such. Your body will have developed a dependency on carbs as its source of energy. When you provide it with new foods, it will not expect it. Although it would be ideal for you to have a perfect solution to this, you will just have to power through this stage. Your body will eventually get used to the new foods and will even develop a dependency on them. You may experience a variety of symptoms at first. You will be tired and feel drained of energy. Your skin may break out. You may feel stressed, anxious, and depressed. You may even lose motivation. Although these are not fun, it is entirely worth it. You must keep motivating yourself to get through this phase. You must constantly remind yourself of why you're doing this; it's for your health. Your body will be so much better off once you become adjusted to this diet. In the meantime, however, you will have to go through this phase.

There are ways to make the first few weeks easier and some steps that you definitely should take. You must take some action beforehand. Do some research and decide the proper portions and nutrients that you must get. Speak to a medical professional. Once you do that, you can come up with a plan of action. Perhaps you can make a list of all of the foods and meals that you would like to eat while on the diet. This will help you to stay motivated. By reminding yourself of all of the wonderful foods that there are to eat while on the diet, you will help yourself to become excited about the diet. Although it isn't possible for everyone, it would help to gradually ease into the diet instead of jumping into it cold.

This will help you and your body to slowly adjust. Perhaps consider switching out all bread for lettuce wraps at first. Instead of wheat pasta, choose zucchini pasta. These little switches will help your body to adjust and will reduce the symptoms that you experience during the adjustment period. However, you must come up with a proper plan if you choose this way. Identify all of the foods in your diet that need to be cut out or replaced, and have a written, week-by-week plan for what you will start eating and when. Otherwise, you may become comfortable with where you are and stop making progress. For some people, however, a partial diet is enough. If you are only trying to improve slightly, then maybe this is enough for you.

However, you will most certainly not experience all of the benefits of the alkaline diet unless you fully follow the diet. But you must also make sure that the goals you set for yourself are realistic. Often, people go into diets too quickly without adjusting and it's too much for them. Perhaps French fries make you really happy and you don't want to live with them. Maybe then you can consider having them on special occasions. You must do what's right for you. However, you must also keep in mind that you won't experience the full benefits of the diet if you are still consuming junk.

Overall, you must remember to properly transition and keep your goals in mind. It will be tough, but it's worth it. You are working towards improving your health. After the first few weeks, you will have adjusted and will feel so much better. You will experience all of the benefits of the diet and will lower your risk for the detriments of an unhealthy diet.

Cravings

You will get cravings of the old foods that you used to consume. This is the harsh truth. It's inevitable. When you go from eating these foods often to completely cutting them out, your body will want them. The other harsh truth is that junk food is tasty. It's enjoyable to eat. You must combat these cravings, however, because your body receives nothing but negative reactions from consuming these foods. They are not helpful to your health. There are ways to combat these cravings, though. It may take time for them to subside, but it will require work in the meantime. There are some tips and tricks for avoiding cravings and combatting them.

It is important that you designate specific times of the day to eat. It is recommended to have a few smaller meals throughout the day instead of a couple of big meals a day, but it is up to you and what your doctor recommends for you. If you are not eating often enough or not eating enough during your meals, you will face hunger. When you're hungry, your body will want whatever food it can get, and your logic will be impaired, leading to possible consumption of unhealthy foods. It is wise to plan out when each meal or snack is.

This will allow you to feed your body when it needs it. You shouldn't ever go five hours or more without food (when you are awake), as your blood sugar levels will drop, and you will be hungry. Have snacks available to you at all times that will keep you going and reduce your hunger. It is wise to keep dried fruit in the car, food at work, and make sure to eat before you leave the house. This will help you to not be as hungry.

It is also important for you to eat protein. Protein keeps you full for longer, which will also help you to not be as hungry. Nuts are a great source of protein, and they are very easy to bring with you wherever you go. When you eat something sugary such as fruit, you will get short-term energy. This will provide you with energy for a small period of time, and then you will "crash." Protein is a long-term source of protein and will keep you full for an extended period of time.

It is also important to stay hydrated. What often happens is that your body thinks it's hungry, but you are actually dehydrated. For many, this feeling is the same. Your stomach will feel empty, and you feel like you need to consume something. If you drink water throughout the day, you won't experience this feeling as often. Your cravings for salty foods will also be lowered. When you are dehydrated, your body will want salty foods. Keep some water with you at all times, and make sure that you are constantly drinking. This will also help you to stay hydrated, which is an added bonus.

For cravings of food that your body misses, you can try distracting yourself. Try going out, talking to a friend, or doing something that you love. This can help your brain to be happy and satisfied without caving into any of those unhealthy food +cravings. Sometimes, people crave food simply because they are bored. You may also crave it to cure some sort of negative emotion that you are feeling. By choosing a healthier way to cope with those feelings, you are helping your body to be healthier. Depending on food for curing unideal emotions is not a healthy way to cope with problems. You may try being active, doing a hobby of yours, or talking to people. When in doubt, brush your teeth. You won't want to eat anything afterward, because it will all taste bad. You also won't want to mess up how clean and fresh you just made your mouth.

Cravings can arise both physically and mentally. When you become physically dependent on food, your body becomes addicted to it. The more you eat, the more you will want of it. Cutting out a portion of food that your body has become addicted to can make your body "need" it. When you don't give it to your body, it will want you to consume it so that it can be satisfied. Mental cravings result from the desire of a certain food. Perhaps it tastes good. Regardless, cravings of unhealthy foods can and should be combatted.

Social Eating and Drinking

Eating and drinking have become highly social events. When humans first roamed the Earth, eating was a reward for the task of gathering the food. It was what kept them alive. Now, eating is a fun event. There are restaurants that will serve you. There are countless options for snacks, meals, and drinks. Every day, companies release new flavors and food products. The options for eating seem to never end. Additionally, eating has become a social event. Friends, family, and business partners invite each other over for dinner, eat out at restaurants, and enjoy ice cream cones together. It seems that there is a social culture built around eating. Holidays are days for eating and drinking. It seems that there is always some excuse for eating a large amount of junk food. It is used for celebration, to alleviate emotional pain, and for fun.

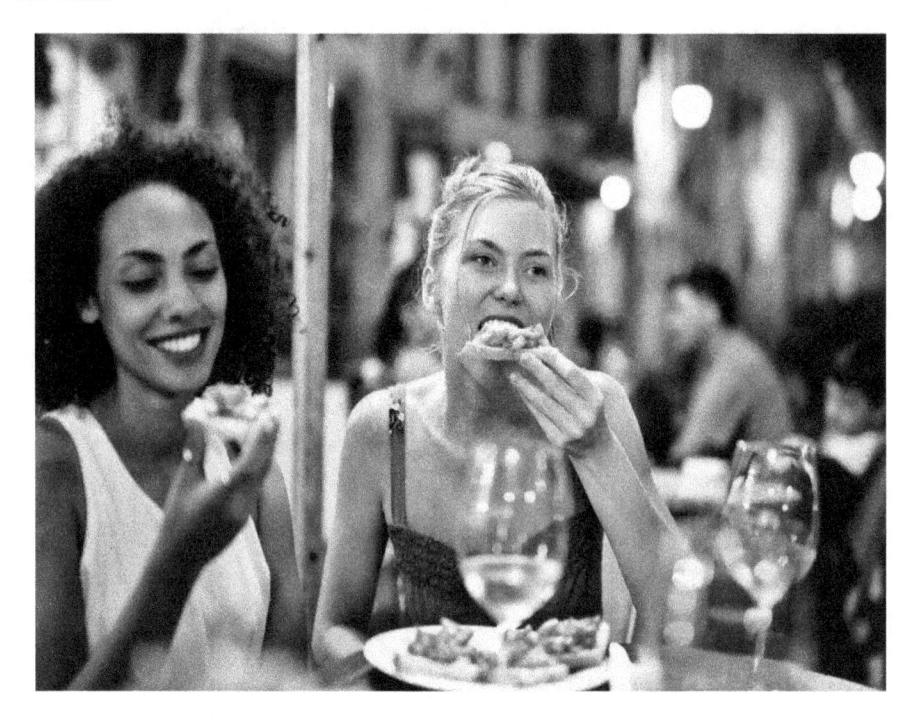

So, how do you break this habit?

Social eating is difficult because what will often happen is that you won't be able to eat most of the food that is at the event. You most likely won't want to say no, either. Yet when going to eat with friends, there will probably always be some sort of option that will be okay for your diet. You don't have to completely cut out all socializing because of your diet. That will just leave you miserable. When going to a restaurant, get a salad without the dressing. Perhaps you can get some side dishes of fruits or vegetables.

When eating at someone's house, look for options that will work for you. You can still enjoy the event without eating one of everything. If someone asks you to try something that falls out of your diet, politely tell them that you are on a diet and thank them for offering it to you. People aren't going to lose respect for you or dislike you because you didn't get a slice of the triple chocolate cake.

They may actually respect you more because you have self-control and care about what you are putting into your body. Although there may be pressure for having "seconds" or filling up your plate, stay aware of your portion sizes. You don't need to overeat or stuff yourself. Stay aware of your body, and don't eat past the point of fullness.

It may help to eat beforehand. That way, you won't be tempted to shove the nearest food into your mouth. You won't mindlessly eat unhealthy foods. It will help you to maintain your logic. This is similar to the idea of never grocery shopping while hungry. You will be more inclined to pick up unhealthy foods that you otherwise wouldn't, and you will be more likely to pick out items that you won't actually eat.

Be sure that your focus isn't on food. Talk to people. Socialize instead of eating the whole time. It may help to distance yourself from where the food is. If you are in constant view of the food and people eating it, you will be tempted to do the same. Make sure you drink lots of water the whole time. Plan beforehand to not overeat and don't feel guilty for not finishing your food or eating as much as other people are. Nobody will be upset with you for doing so, and you will feel better.

You must also get over social drinking. In college, many parties are centered around drinking excessively. Some people never get over that. Others drink occasionally during holidays and events. It is seen as "mature" and "professional" to drink and serve wine. However, it is only beneficial to stop drinking. Drinking can inhibit your physical and cognitive functions, which can be very dangerous, especially if you are driving. It can be harmful to you and your health. Alcohol is very unhealthy for your liver.

When out at a social event that involves drinking, it is okay to refuse the offer to drink. You can say no and drink water. You will still have a good time and enjoy the same things. People won't stop liking you just because you don't drink. Prepare a response for when someone offers you a drink. It is okay to say no. If you feel better without drinking, that is reason alone to not do it. Hangovers can hinder productivity the next day and hold you back. People will respect you for your decision. If they don't, they are not good people to be surrounding yourself with. There is much more to life than drinking. It is also always good to be fully aware of your body and actions.

Social eating and drinking may be hard to resist at first, but you will feel much better and be able to easily avoid the temptations of each.

Portion Control and Getting Enough Nutrients

For many, portion control is difficult. With social pressure and large portion sizes at restaurants, it seems as if we are being trained to eat more and more. You must make sure that you are eating enough to fuel your body, but you also must ensure that you are not eating too much. When you are on a plant-based diet, it will take more of those foods to equal the same amount of fuel that a calorie-rich food such as meat will give you. The foods are less densely packed with calories and fat. This means that you can eat too little because you are not used to having to eat so much. It can also mean that you can overcompensate and eat too much as a result. Finding that balance is important.

Even if you are eating the right foods, you must be eating the right amount of them to truly maximize your health. Too much of a good thing is not always a good problem to have. Some foods are easy to overindulge on. Almonds and nuts contain a lot of fat and protein, and they are easy to snack on. If you mindlessly eat them, you will be putting more protein and fat into your body that is healthy.

You are also setting yourself up for a bad habit. When you overeat constantly, your body will have trouble digesting so much food. You will feel worn out as a result. This can also cause you to gain weight and have an unhealthy relationship with food. It may even lead to an eating disorder. It is not at all healthy to binge on food. If you can't stop yourself from eating, especially when you are full, you will have a very unhealthy relationship with food and will struggle mentally as a result.

To avoid overeating, it may help to drink water before your meal. You can also dine on smaller plates to make it seem like you are eating more than you are, and you won't feel guilty about not filling up your plate. Also, be sure to properly portion your food. Never eat straight from the bag. Put your food on a separate plate and make sure that you put the right amount out. Eat slowly so that your stomach has time to register what you are putting into it. This will also help you to enjoy your food more. Mindlessly eating while being unaware of your portions can lead to serious health problems and a bad relationship with food.

You must also be sure that you are eating enough. Because you are on a plant-based diet, you won't realize how much your body needs until you become aware of it. On a meat-based diet, you are quickly filled because the foods are densely packed with calories. However, it would take much more fruit and vegetables to give you the same amount of energy. There are many plant-based foods that will still give you the calories and energy that you need, however. Nuts, oils, and avocado will help you to reach your caloric goals. Make sure that you are getting enough protein, fat, and calories. It is wise to speak with your doctor or another medical professional before starting the diet so that you can ensure that you are getting exactly the amount that you need to function properly and stay healthy. These amounts will completely depend on the person, as they vary based on your weight, height, age, gender, activity level, genetics, and possible health conditions. Make sure that you plan your meals with this in mind. You must conduct your research beforehand to make sure that you are getting what you need. It may help to get a mobile app that can help you track your food, its calories, and its macronutrients. It is important to stay healthy and balanced.

There are several foods that can help you to reach your goals in protein, fat, and calories. You may eat nuts such as almonds, cashews, walnuts, and pecans. These are great for snacks and adding to meals. Avocado is also rich in fat and calories and can be added to smoothies, salads, and (lettuce) wraps. Quinoa has calories and protein, and it is great as a side, in soup, and in salads. Olive oil has fat and calories, and it can be added to salads or with vegetables to add flavor. Dried fruit is great. The water has been taken out of the fruit, which allows you to have fruit that is more concentrated than the original. Beans and chickpeas are great, and they can be added to a variety of dishes. The sweet potato is a vegetable that is rich in calories. Smoothies help you to mix a bunch of ingredients at once, allowing you to get more calories packed into a single drink. Wild rice is alkaline diet-approved and can serve as a side or as an addition to a meal. Coconut oil is rich in fat and can be mixed in with smoothies and salads.

While on a plant-based diet, it is important that you don't become deficient in any nutrients. A nutrient deficiency can lead to serious health problems. It is quite common for those who switch to plant-based diets to develop deficiencies simply because they are unaware that they exist. There are certain nutrients that are found in meat that simply aren't as common or plentiful in plant-based foods. If you make yourself aware of these beforehand, however, you can be prepared and prevent this from happening to you.

Anemia occurs when you are deficient in vitamin B12. This issue causes your body to be low in red blood cells, which can cause circulation and respiration problems. It can cause a variety of health problems. Many on plant-based diets choose to take a supplement of vitamin B12 to avoid this deficiency.

Vitamin D deficiency is a common deficiency to have, yet it can easily be fixed by subjecting yourself to sun exposure. Make sure that you put on sunscreen, though! Omega-3 fatty acids are common to be deficient in, yet they can be found in seeds and nuts. Zinc is another deficiency that is common with those on a plant-based diet, yet it can be found in beans and legumes. Iron is yet another common deficiency, and it may be found in leafy greens, whole grains, peas, and dried fruit.

You must take care of your body properly. Adjusting to a diet will be hard. You will have to get used to eat, avoid social pressure with eating and drinking, combat cravings, and make sure that you are eating the right amount and aren't deficient in any nutrients. You must take care of your body because it is the only one that you have.

Chapter 9

Tips and Tricks

Starting a new diet is tough! It can be difficult to start a new habit and maintain it. It's important that you surround yourself with good influences. It will also help you to prepare your meals beforehand so that you can be sure of exactly what it is that you are eating and that you are receiving enough food. There are also some further tricks beyond dieting to make sure that you are maximizing your health. The alkaline diet is really great for your health!

Ways to Maintain the Habit

There are many tips to help you to have an easier time maintaining your diet. It will be difficult, but there are ways to make it much easier for yourself and to help you stick to the diet. It is important to power through the tough times and makes sure that you are setting realistic goals for yourself.

It is important to reward yourself and not punish yourself. When starting a new habit, it is very likely that you will mess up, especially at first. You may cave into cravings. You may not treat your body properly. You may suffer symptoms of transitioning into a new diet. However, it is important to never punish yourself. You are on a journey to improve your health. Beating yourself up won't fix the food that you shouldn't have eaten. It won't solve your problems. As long as you are constantly improving yourself and your health, you are doing a great job. Every little bit counts. By beating yourself up, you may become unmotivated and slip into poor habits again. Instead, reward yourself. Set goals every week. When you accomplish these goals, celebrate. Perhaps you love taking baths or have been eyeing something that you want to buy. Go out with friends and have a good time. Rewarding yourself will encourage you to accomplish even more.

It is really helpful to have a buddy that can help push you further. Try to recruit a friend or family member to do the diet with you. By having someone to talk to, it will be much easier to stick to the diet. You also won't feel alone in what you are doing. You will have someone that will hold you accountable for sticking to the diet, and you will also have someone to celebrate your success with. There are many online communities for those who are on plant-based diets. It is worth it to check it out and make friends with people who are on the same track as you. You can share recipes, experiences, and tips with each other. You may even decide to cook for one another. Having a community of people to surround yourself with that have the same goals as you is very motivating.

It is also helpful to track your meals. There are many mobile apps that allow you to enter in the food that you ate and will tell you the number of calories, fat, and other nutrients that are in it. This can help you to keep track of if you are getting all of the nutrients you need. It can also help you to track your portion sizes.

One more way of helping you to maintain your diet is to start journaling. This is a great way to document how you feel and let it all out. It is also helpful to see how your body reacts to certain foods. This is especially helpful for the first few weeks that you are adjusting to the new food, as you will be able to write down exactly how it is that you feel.

Meal Prepping

Meal prepping is a great way to maintain your diet properly. This will allow you to effectively prepare your meals and properly portion them. It can also allow you to have meals that are ready to go so that you aren't tempted to get fast food or the like. It is helpful to get reusable containers and set up meals for the entire week ahead. This is actually faster because you only have to make the food at one time instead of spreading it out.

It can help you to reduce the stress about preparing meals. You won't have to rush around at the last minute to throw a meal together for yourself. You will also reduce cravings. With meal prepping, you are making the food ahead of time and won't be hungry; you will have food made for yourself and already planned out. You can plan your meals to have the perfect amount of everything. They will be portioned properly and contain the right amount of nutrients in them. It also saves money. Instead of eating out, you can have all of your meals made from home. You also won't be as tempted to eat out because you prepared food for yourself already. You can also buy in bulk and you won't be wasting your money. You will use exactly what you need, and you won't feel the need to buy unnecessary items for yourself. There will actually be a plan instead of having chaos associated with your meals. You may also completely customize it to fit your needs. You can prepare meals that you like and that work for you. It also makes it easier for you to eat foods that comply with your diet. It just makes sense to meal prep. It is the easier, healthier, and cheaper way to eat.

An Overall Healthier You

Diet isn't the only influence on your health. You must take care of all of the aspects of your life in order to be healthy. As far as physical health goes, diet is only half of the problem. You must also ensure that you are staying active and exercising enough. You must care for your mental and emotional health. Your space should be clutter-free and calming to you. You must ensure that you have some sort of hobby to allow yourself to be creative and remain happy. Journaling and meditating are common ways to maintain your mental health. You must also ensure that your relationships with friends and family are healthy. Otherwise, you will not be happy. Diet isn't the only aspect of your health. However, it is a way to lead to greater health and start the journey of being your happiest and healthiest self. Dieting can help you to consume the proper foods, which will give you more energy and motivate you to keep the other aspects of your health in check. It is important to take care of your body so that you are the happiest and healthiest that you can be.

It is crucial to stay active. Luckily, a proper diet will help with this. You will be able to have the energy to get out and be active. It is important to have cardio, strength, and flexibility exercises in your routine to ensure maximum health. Cardio exercises are great for strengthening your heart health. Strength exercises will help your muscles and bones to be stronger. Flexibility will help you to regain your balance and will help your mental health. It is important to stay active every day. You don't have to intensely work out every day, but make sure that you are moving. Take a walk, ride your bike, or go swimming. There are many easy ways to stay active. It is also helpful to always push yourself and improve your activity level.

You must also practice self-care. Brush your teeth and floss every day. Shower regularly. These are simple tasks that seem like no-brainers to most, yet they are very important for your health. It is important to regularly visit both the doctor and the dentist purely to check up on your health and make sure that you are doing well. Doing so is crucial. It is much better to catch any health problems while they can still be fixed, as opposed to after it is too late.

In addition to keeping yourself clean, it is important to keep your surroundings clean. This will reduce stress and allow you to be productive. If you have many items in your work environment that are cluttered, your thoughts will be cluttered as well. If you have any items that are weighing you down, need attention, or that you feel guilty about, you need to act. Items like these will cause you unnecessary stress and bring down other aspects of your health.

Take steps to maximize your mental health. It is important to balance the time that you spend with your friends, family, and yourself. You must also ensure that the people you surround yourself with are right. They must be motivating and supportive, and they shouldn't pressure you into doing what you don't want to do. Make sure that you maintain good relationships with those in your life, including yourself. It is important to have a hobby for yourself to allow you to have time to think and not stress. Common hobbies of this sort include journaling, meditating, and doing yoga. However, there are many ways to keep peace in your life. Being active is perfect because you are having time to yourself and staying active. Reading and listening to music are other peaceful activities that can help you. If you have a creative hobby such as photography, knitting, or painting, these are great ways to express yourself and keep your mental health up. It is important to take care of your health, both mentally and physically. This will allow you to maximize your health and the benefits of the alkaline diet. It will also help you to be a much happier person overall, and you will enjoy life much more.

Overall, the alkaline diet is not too difficult. There are ways to make it easier for yourself. It can be simple to maintain the habit. It really helps to have someone that can accompany you on your journey to better health. You must also remember to keep all aspects of your health in check. In doing so, you are really helping yourself.

Conclusion

Now you know everything that you need to know about the alkaline diet. You learned all about the alkaline diet and the science behind it. You learned what you must be careful of before starting and while on the diet. You also learned about the microbiome and how microbes affect your body and serve a large role in your health. Also talked about were the three golden keys. You must reset your body, rebalance it, and reconnect with it. These are important steps to transitioning to the alkaline diet. There are also a number of acid-producing foods and habits that you should avoid in order to maximize your health. It is also important to know how exactly the alkaline diet is beneficial for you, your body, and your health. There are many alkaline-promoting foods and meals that are able to be enjoyed ensuring that you follow the diet and that you have a broad selection of foods and drinks to choose from. Because diets are difficult to start and stick to, there are also quite a few troubleshooting tricks to make sure that you can follow the diet and still maintain good health. Tips and tricks are also provided to help you to know how to properly stick to the diet. Overall, the alkaline diet is highly beneficial for your health. However, it is always important to familiarize yourself with the science behind a diet before committing to one. This will ensure that you are properly educated on the right way to treat your body. It will also ensure that you are able to take care of yourself properly.

Alkaline Diet Cookbook

Easy and Quick Alkaline Recipes, Natural Weight Loss for Massive Energy, Prevent and Reverse Disease through Alkaline Foods and Herbal Healing. 10 Day Meal Plan

Introduction

Congratulations on downloading *Alkaline Diet Cookbook* and thank you for doing so.

The following chapters will discuss all the things that you need to know in order to get started on the alkaline diet! There are a lot of different options to choose from when it is time to work with a diet plan to improve their health, but none are going to focus on your body and the way it works the way that the alkaline diet does. We will take some time to explore how this works and the steps that you need to know to help you see some great results.

To start, we are going to take a look at some of the basics that come with the alkaline diet plan. We will look at what this plan is all about, why it is effective, why the pH levels in your body are so important (along with why you should keep an eye on them and how to check them), and some other factors that will make the alkaline diet a bit easier to focus on and do well with.

Once we have a good understanding of the alkaline diet plan, it is time to move on to some of the rules about eating on this diet plan. In this chapter, we are going to explore some of the foods that are alkaline and are highly encouraged, and some of the foods that are seen as more acidic and should be avoided. We will also bring in the topic of alkaline water and how this can be beneficial to get the most out of this diet plan.

From this point, we will spend some time looking at the different foods that you are able to consume when you are on the alkaline diet. We will look at a 10-day meal plan along with some delicious foods and recipes that are going to work well for those who are trying to find meals for breakfast, lunch, dinner, snacks, desserts, and more while on this diet plan.

Sometimes, the hardest part of getting started on a new diet plan, especially one like the alkaline diet, is finding the foods that you need to consume to make it work. This part of the guidebook, along with the bonus chapter about alkaline friendly herbs, will make this part a bit easier. You will be ready to go through your first ten days on the alkaline diet, with the meals and the recipes all planned out for you!

When it comes to going on a diet plan and trying to find ways to improve your health and help you to feel better in no time at all, there is nothing that is better than going on the alkaline diet plan. When you are ready to learn a bit more about this diet plan and how it can work for you, make sure to check out this guidebook to help you get started!

There are plenty of books on this subject on the market, thanks again for choosing this one! Every effort was made to ensure it is full of as much useful information as possible. Please enjoy!

Chapter 1

What is the Alkaline Diet?

Going on a diet plan to improve your health and make you feel as amazing as possible can be hard. You want to make sure that you are picking out the right one, the one that is going to improve or prevent a variety of health conditions and even helps you to lose weight along the way. You also want to make sure that the diet plan is going to be healthy, and that you won't put in the hard work to see that nothing is going to happen for you.

The alkaline diet is going to be a bit different than what we see with some of the other diet plans that are out there. While many of those can be healthy for you, and promote all of the weight that you could potentially lose, the alkaline diet is going to focus more on the health component of the diet plan. Sure, when you switch away from some of the foods that are known as acidic and focus more on foods that are healthy and wholesome for you, it is so much easier for you to lose weight. But the main goal here is to learn what raises the acidity in your body and what will lower it. Once we know that, we can gain control over all of our health needs.

This chapter is going to help us look a bit more closely at the alkaline diet and all that it is able to provide to us in terms of our health. Some of the things that you need to know about the alkaline diet include:

The Basics of the Alkaline Diet

Before we get too far into some of the recipes that come with the alkaline diet, we need first to get a better understanding of what this diet plan is all about. The idea behind this kind of plan is that you will learn how to consume the foods that will help your body to balance out its pH value. The pH value is a measurement of the balance between acidity and alkalinity in your body. Your goal is to keep these numbers balanced and level as much as possible to help keep your health up and running well.

Your metabolism, which is simply the process of the body taking the food you eat and converting it to the energy you can use, is sometimes seen as a type of fire. It is going to have some chemical reactions found inside that are able to break down any solid mass that you are working with. However, these chemical reactions are usually going to happen at a slower rate than a real fire, but they are still important.

As your metabolism does its work, it is going to leave a bit of waste or residue behind it. The acid from your food can either be acidic, alkaline, or neutral based on what you consume. To keep things simple, if you end up eating a lot of foods over the long term that are more acidic, the acidic ash is going to turn your blood this way as well. But if you eat foods that can leave behind alkaline ash, the opposite will be true.

When we take a look at this idea, we see that there are some foods that are going to be acidic and foods that are going to be seen as more alkaline. Learning which ones fit into each category will be important to improving your overall health.

While the majority of this plan is going to focus on the foods that are acidic that you need to avoid and the foods that are more alkaline that you are allowed to have in abundance, there are other factors that can come into play to help balance out the pH levels in the body. For example, getting enough sleep, reducing the amount of stress you feel in your life, and exercising can all work together with the various foods that you decide to consume in order to change up the pH levels in the body.

What is pH and why is it important?

One of the things that we concentrate on quite a bit when it comes to the alkaline diet is the idea of pH and why it is so important to keeping us as healthy as possible. There are a lot of diet plans that miss out on this important part of your health, and that is why it is sometimes hard to follow them and lose weight or improve your overall health. Learning about pH and how it is going to affect your overall health can make a big difference in how you understand the alkaline diet.

The balance in the body between the alkalinity and the acidity is going to be known as the pH or the potential of hydrogen. There are going to be a lot of different factors that come into play that help determine whether the blood is going to contain too little or too much acid, and one of these things is the food you eat and how healthy your organs are. Being able to achieve the right pH levels can take some work, but you will find that healthy eating habits will make a world of difference with this one.

The level of the pH of your body is going to range from a scale of 0 to 14. The lower the pH, the more acidic your body is, and the higher the pH, the more alkaline. Your body is neutral when it reaches a pH of 7.0, which is going to be the same pH as water. The optimal pH for your body to stay healthy and not have too much acid inside is going to be somewhere around 7.45 or slightly lower. If you allow it to get too far over to the other side of things, then you are going to end up with too much acid in the body, your organs and your health will start to notice.

You will find that there are a lot of health conditions that will be linked back to the amount of acid that is found in the body. The more acid that is there and the longer it is allowed to stay around, the worse your health is going to be. If you are suffering from obesity, heart problems, diabetes, IBS, and other conditions, especially if there is more than one of these in your health charts, then it may be time to make some changes to get your health back on track. And lowering your body acid levels and changing them to be more alkaline is a great way to get started.

As we explore with the alkaline diet, the foods that you eat can really make a difference in how alkaline and how acidic your body is going to be. There are some foods that are higher in acid, and it is best to limit them as much as possible. This would include foods like cheese, beef, walnuts, chocolate, blackberries, and prunes.

The good news is there are also some foods that are able to help the body reach a more alkaline state. These can include foods like olive oil, spinach, asparagus, and watermelon, to name a few. Making sure that you eat foods that are well balanced and includes lots of fruits and vegetables and plenty of variety is a great way to ensure that you take care of your health while also balancing out your pH levels in the process.

Microbiomes and What Role They Play In Alkalinity

The next thing that we are going to take a look at here is the idea of the microbiome. The body of a human is a really complex system. One of the places where our bodies are able to interact quite a bit with the outside world is our gut. The stomach is going to be the frontline when it comes to the immune system, and it is going to be exposed all of the time to new molecules and microbes that results from all of the foods that the body consumes.

The brain, located in the central nervous system, is where you can see some of these processes happening, which may somehow influence the people's mood a little bit. But it is important to take a closer look at some of the organisms that are found there to determine what they do to keep the stomach, and the body, up and running.

From here, we need to explore what a microbiome is. Microbiota is referred to the collection of microbiomes that can be found living inside and on the body of a human being. Inside the microbes, you can find the genes called the microbiome. These genes are important because they are going to be able to influence how the body is going to operate on a day to day basis. And these genes are so prevalent that they are able to outnumber the human genes with a 100:1 ratio.

The neat thing here is that we all are going to have unique microbiomes and microbiota. What you expose your body into will determine the microbes that live in there. You will also find that they always change. Things that are able to change the genes of these microbes include your gender, age, diet, stress, health status, and even where you live.

Scientists already know about these microorganisms for centuries. The discovery of tiny animalcules, found using a microscope, was already written in 1673 by Antony van Leeuwenhoek. Leeuwenhoek was amazed because he was able to find these microbes in almost any place that he tried to look, but the sad thing is that the society often ignored these discoveries until almost the 1900s when their function in the spread, and even the cause of disease, was found.

While microbes can play a role in our health and can be a spread of disease when bacteria and others get into the body, the microbe is something that is already found in us, and we have our own unique set that helps to determine how the body will function.

It is believed that humans are going to carry bacteria of almost 3 pounds in their stomachs. The microbiome that you have in your body is going to be as unique as your fingerprints, and it will not match what someone else is going to have for their own. And each of these microbiomes will have many various types of bacteria, though the amount of these will vary from day to day depending on the kinds of situations the person finds themselves in at any given time.

The role of the microbiome is going to be very important to the operations of the body, and it can pretty much act as its own organ. And when the microbiome is working in the proper manner, it is going to help impact things like cognitive function, mood, the immune system, digestion, and aging. When it is not working well, all of these things are going to start suffering.

Some of the bacteria that we have in the stomach are able to come in and produce some enzymes that help us with digestion. These bacteria are also going to provide us with short chain fatty acids, vitamin K, and the B vitamins as well. The microbiota also influences the metabolic rate in the body.

We want to have a strong amount of microbiome in the body because, in addition to aiding with digestion, it is going to be the foundation of how well our immune system is able to work. When we were first born, the gut is as clean as a slate ready to be filled with new experiences. Exposure to microbes is going to provide the education needed to train our immune system how to respond to various organisms and more that may sneak in. Because of this, the immune system is going to mediate the relationship between the body and the microbes that it hosts. The harmful organisms can be dealt with, the helpful ones will get to stay and help contribute to your good health if the system is working properly.

The problem is that when we eat foods that are hard on the body, all of the processed and sugary junk that we just don't need, we find that we are not going to be helping those microbiomes do their job. They are going to get damaged and run into some problems along the way as well.

Once these are damaged, we are going to start to notice. We will not be able to absorb the nutrients from our diets in the manner that we should. We will not be able to fight off infections because that critical tie between our stomachs and the immune system is damaged and perhaps even broken over time. And the longer that we continue to stick with foods that are acidic and damaging to our health, the more ill health and other conditions we are going to face.

This is where the alkaline diet can come into play. It is going to ensure that you can repair the microbiome and other parts of the body in the process. It is a simple solution to changing up your diet plan without having to go through and really harm yourself with bad medications and more. Just by changing up some of the foods that you eat and learning how to limit and eliminate some of the foods that are seen as bad, you will be able to get your health back on track and get those microbiomes to start doing their jobs again.

These microbiomes are so important to your overall health. When they are working well thanks to your alkaline diet, you will notice a difference. Your body will be able to take in the nutrients that you consume easier, you will have more energy, and your immune system will finally be able to do the work that it needs to fight off infections and illnesses in a way that medications and surgeries just are not able to do. Making it your goal to eat right and work on enhancing those microbiomes in the body is the first step to getting your overall health back in line.

Why does my body need to be alkaline?

There are a lot of different reasons why your body needs to be more alkaline and less acidic. Basically, when your body is acidic, it is opening the door for a lot of illness and disease to spread. These diseases love to be in an environment that is highly acidic, one that isn't alkaline at all, because this is exactly what they need to stay healthy along the way.

When you eat foods that raise the acid levels in the body, you will find that you get sick more often, you get more infections, your energy levels are lower, and a whole host of other conditions along the way. This is a problem that a lot of Americans are dealing with because of their poor food choices, and it is part of why they are getting so sick so often.

By changing the pH levels in the body around a bit, you will find that you can fight off the infections, the diseases, and more. These things are not able to survive in an environment that is alkaline. So, just by turning the body slightly alkaline, or even neutral, may be just what you need to help get yourself in the best health possible.

The alkaline diet is going to help you to get this all done. It is responsible for teaching us the best things to do to cut out some of the acidity in the body and get healthier. By learning the right goods to consume on this diet and which ones that you need to limit if not eliminate, you will be able to change up the pH levels in the body to something that the illnesses and the diseases just are not able to survive in!

There is so much good that you can get out of going on the alkaline diet plan. It is one of the best options to choose because it is simple, and it ensures that we are going to see some great health benefits along the way. It may take some time to adjust to, and learning how to give up some acidic foods that may have been our favorites in the past can be hard in the beginning. But overall, it is well worth our time to learn more about the alkaline diet and to learn how to follow some of the rules that come with it.

Chapter 2

The Benefits of the Alkaline Diet

The next thing that we are going to take a look at is some of the health benefits that you are able to enjoy when it comes to working with the alkaline diet. When you are looking into this kind of diet plan, one of the things that you may show some interest in is the different health benefits of this plan. The cool thing is that there are a lot of health benefits, even more than you are able to see with some traditional forms of dieting that are so popular right now.

Whether you have dealt with health conditions like diabetes, cancer, heart disease, skin redness, hair loss, and more, you will find that the alkaline diet is going to be the best option to help keep you healthy. There are so many ways that are simply balancing out your pH levels and taking care of yourself with the right foods and avoiding the wrong foods can benefit the whole body. Some of the different health benefits that you are going to be able to enjoy when you go on this kind of diet plan include:

Great at Fighting off Diabetes

Many Americans are going to deal with diabetes at one point or another. There are so many different factors that are found in the traditional diet that most Americans eat that can lead us to develop diabetes. But when we decide to go with the alkaline diet, you will find that it is easier to decrease the issues with diabetes, helping to fight it off better than any other method or even prevent it in the first place.

With the traditional American diet, you are going to end up with lots of sugars and processed carbs. Many people eat processed foods, easy to make meals, sweets, and more that are going to be loaded with these carbs and sugars. The body is not able to use all of these, and that results in problems with insulin resistance and trying to move those nutrients out of the body. If the problem goes on for too long, it is going to end up with the body not knowing how to handle the insulin that it receives or the carbs and sugars, and then diabetes ensues.

But with the alkaline diet, you are learning how to limit and even eliminate some of these foods that are going to cause diabetes. You will still eat some healthy carbs, and you will still get a bit of sugar from the fruits that you eat. But the amounts are much lower. Plus, these carbs and sugars are different and much healthier than the ones that you were eating in the past.

When you are able to focus on the healthy sugars and carbs, while eliminating the ones that may be pretty bad for you, you will find it is much easier to reduce your risk of diabetes and even get any current problems with diabetes that you have!

Helps you to go Through a Detox

The neat thing about adding in so many healthy foods into the diet that you are on is that you are then able to give the body everything that it needs, from minerals and vitamins, without all of the bad stuff. This is something that you need to focus on when it is time to rid the body of acid, and you want to go through a natural detox that will improve so many aspects of your overall health.

For those of us who have been following a traditional American diet for a long time, it is highly likely that your body is looking for a good detox to help it out. This is sometimes hard to trust in and get started with because we aren't sure How to make: the detox start and works for us. But simply by going on the alkaline diet and focusing on the foods that are allowed in this diet plan, and avoiding, as much as possible the acidic foods out there, you will find that you will be able to give the body the detox that it needs.

This Diet can Help to Improve the Health of your Brain

There are going to be a lot of different ways that you are able to work with the alkaline diet in order to improve the health of your brain, something that other diet plans may not be able to do. First, many of those who decide to go on this diet plan are going to see that just going with the eating plan will provide the brain with more of the healthy nutrients that it needs to stay in the best health possible, while helping you to think critically, helps with the memory, reduces brain fog, and so much more.

First, when you learn how to eliminate some of the foods that are bad for the brain, such as carbs, sugars, and all processed and junk foods, you are clearing out the mind. Sure, those foods are able to provide you with a quick jolt of energy, but basically, they are going to cause a lot of issues with clouding out the brain and making you feel miserable. When you are able to limit and even eliminate these kinds of foods, your brain is going to be able to stay clear and will focus more than before.

Another benefit is that you are going to start taking in so many good nutrients that are going to enhance your brain functioning as well. You will find that when you eat all of the healthy and wholesome nutrients in that fresh produce that is encouraged on this diet, your health is going to increase, and your brain will see the benefits as well.

Can Help to Lower Inflammation

Many times, when we take a look at the alkaline diet, we are going to also hear about the anti-inflammatory diet. If you have heard about this second diet plan, then you know that inflammation is going to be a huge problem that can just compound over time. Inflammation is going to be uncomfortable and can lead to many of the illnesses, diseases, and pain in the whole body. It is common that people are not going to realize a lot of the common issues they deal with are linked back to the inflammation, and they may not do anything about it until arthritis, and other joint pain starts to be a problem. But when this happens, it is highly likely that the inflammation has spread through the body for a long time, and the person just didn't feel it or realize.

It is true that a bit of inflammation through the body on occasion is not a bad thing. Inflammation is a natural response of the body to heal itself after a cut or when you get sick or an infection. But the inflammation that we bring up here is going to be different. This inflammation is there for a long time and doesn't go away. And it isn't protecting you or fighting off any illness at all. And this is a big reason why it is going to cause a lot of issues with your health.

One of the biggest benefits that you are going to see when you go on this alkaline diet is that it can help to fight off the chronic inflammation going through your body. You are taking away some of the acids that causes the inflammation, and that results in easier management of pain, the ability to fight off cancer, and even a reduction in the risk you have for developing diabetes.

Helps with Hypertension by Lowering Blood Pressure

The next benefit that we are going to see when we work with the alkaline diet is the fact that the foods that you eat and the ones that you end up eliminating are going to help you to lower your blood pressure. Hypertension and high blood pressure are going to be serious issues that many people in the country are going to be dealing with right now. While it is possible that a bit of it comes from genetics, most are going to come from an unhealthy lifestyle that includes lots of poor diet choices and not enough movement.

The problem is that the longer you allow the high blood pressure to remain, the worse the problem will end up being for you. Learning some healthy ways to handle your hypertension without having to be on a lot of medications that often just mask the problem rather than helping it is what will actually make the difference for you.

When you decide to go on the alkaline diet, you get the benefit of reducing any risk that you have for hypertension. There are a few reasons for this, but one is because it is able to decrease how much inflammation is found in the body. Add in that, the alkaline diet helps with the production of human growth hormone, which is needed to fight off diseases like hypertension, and you will find that your body will respond in a healthier and natural manner including a lowered blood pressure.

See Healthier Teeth and Gums

Just like your body is going to steal some calcium out of the bones when there is too much acid present, it is possible that some of the calcium and minerals from your teeth and gums can be taken as well. But your mouth is going to be more limited on the number of minerals that it is able to share, and this can really cause some issues with the teeth and gums if you are not careful with the acid levels in the body.

The best thing that you can do to handle this kind of problem is to learn how to cut out the acid-forming foods, the ones that are going to really leach out the minerals and calcium from the teeth and gums. And this is exactly what you are going to see happen when you work with the alkaline diet plan.

Can be Great for Weight Loss

Keep in mind with this one that the main goal of the alkaline diet is not to help you lose weight. It is more of a focus on ensuring that you lower the pH levels in the body and get rid of the acid rather than helping you to lose weight. While it stands to reason that if you ate a really poor diet before starting on the alkaline diet, and then you switch over to some of the healthier alternatives in the process, that you would be able to lose weight on this plan as well.

If you are carrying around extra weight that should not be on the body, then this is a big sign that acid is building up in the body as well. In addition to going on an alkaline diet plan that avoids most of the acidic foods out there, there are a few things that you can try to work with in order to get the most out of the alkaline diet, which is going to do wonders when it is time to make the weight fall off your body as well.

First, you should consider adding in some alkaline approved fats to the meals that you eat. You may think that if you want to lose weight, then the fat in your diet needs to be dropped as well. While it may seem a bit strange, it is important to remember that the body needs to have these healthy sources of fat. These fat sources will help the body to absorb and use a lot of the great nutrients and vitamins that you consume through the alkaline diet.

Sticking with lots of healthy fruits and vegetables, a few whole grains, and lean cuts of protein, and maybe a bit of dairy (if you are not intolerant to it) can make a big difference in how you are going to feel on this diet plan. You may also want to experiment with the drinks that you have, opting mainly for alkaline water and green tea most of the time.

Get More Sleep

Another benefit that we are going to take a look at when we explore the alkaline diet is the idea that it can help you to get more sleep. There are many people who, at some point in their lives or another, have had trouble sleeping, suffer from waking up often at night or even waking up in the morning feeling like they tossed and turned so much that they were not able to sleep. If this is something that you are suffering from, then this is a big sign that you are dealing with too much acid in the body. In fact, it is a big sign that the kidneys and the liver are trying to detox the body, but there is just too much acid going on for them to do their jobs.

Your body is often going to be the most acidic when you fall asleep in the middle of the night, even though this may be the opposite of what we would think. And if you are not working on the alkaline diet, the acid is going to get in the way of the detoxing process, and it is going to make sure that you stay wide awake at night. It really gets in the way when you are trying to get some of the healthy and deep REM sleep that the body needs so desperately.

So, this brings up the question of how we are going to make sure that we get enough sleep for the body. One method to use that is approved on the alkaline diet is to eat a lot of green leafy vegetables with your meals. Many of the meals that we provide later in this guidebook will help to fit with this and can make it easier to stick with as well. Options like spinach, kale, broccoli, and more are good at taking some of the acids out of the body and will ensure that you feel better in no time.

After you have gone through and followed the alkaline diet and gotten your body to detox some of the acids that are found in it, you will find that it is so much easier to fall asleep at night, stay asleep, and wake up in the morning feeling refreshed and ready to go. You will wonder why you didn't decide to go on this kind of diet plan earlier thanks to all of the great health benefits that come with it.

More Energy

If you are like many Americans, having enough energy to get through the day is going to be a challenge. You may start your day needing to drink a few cups of coffee, and then by lunchtime or shortly after, you find that you are having a soda or an energy drink or something else that has some caffeine inside of it. And yet you still are dragging and running into issues with having the amount of energy that you need.

One thing to note here is that your energy levels are going to be a big indicator of how healthy you truly are at any given time. When you start to feel tired, one of the first things that you should consider doing even before working with the alkaline diet is taking in some more water. Even adding just a cup or two into your day will provide you with a temporary increase in energy levels. But if you have this and find that the energy leaves quickly, then it may be time to start looking at your diet.

Often, the reason that we are having trouble with our energy supply is because of the foods that we decide to consume. When the majority of your diet consists of sweets, sugars, junk foods, and other processed foods, it is going to cause your energy to go downhill very quickly. They may perk you up a bit, but it will not last long, and you are going to feel your energy levels go down pretty quickly.

When you are able to limit and eliminate some of the bad foods that are listed above, you will find that it makes a huge difference in the amount of energy that you will have. After just a few days, you will notice that you are able to keep up with your life a bit better. You can make it through the day without needing all of the pick-ups like before.

A Reduction in the Amount of Acid Reflux

Right now, it is believed that almost half of Americans are going to suffer from acid reflux to some degree during their lives. Many people believe that this disorder is only going to happen because there is already too much acid around the stomach. This is easy to assume because we think that the reflux is just the acid creeping up through the throat and causing us to feel really uncomfortable in the process as well.

However, this is going to be a false idea. This reflux that we often deal with is going to be caused because the acid in the stomach is lacking. While you want to make sure to eat foods on this diet plan that will help to decrease the amount of acid that you have in your body, you also need to be careful because you want to increase the amount of acid that you are allowing in your stomach.

The trick here is to understand that the acid in the stomach is going to be different compared to the acid in the stomach. The acid in the stomach is completely safe, and it needs to be there so that we can properly digest the food that we eat. The alkaline diet is not going to try and make a reduction in the amount of acid that is in the stomach. It just wants to reduce the acid that is in the rest of the body.

The alkaline diet, the foods that you need to avoid and the ones that you should eat while on this diet plan, will make a big difference in your overall health and can sometimes work to increase the acid that is forming in the stomach to help with reflux. If you find that you are still worried about this and how it is going to work, then you may want to consider adding in a bit of apple cider vinegar to your daily life to help.

Glowing Skin

There are a lot of different skin conditions that you may deal with. Some people find that acne is their issue, but other things like rosacea, eczema, wrinkles, and more can be an issue as well. The thing is, even though these problems seem to have nothing to do with one another, they are all caused by too much acid in the body.

We have to remember that our skin is the biggest organ in the whole body. It needs to receive a lot of nutrition in order to detox and stay as healthy as possible. And when you end up adding too much acid into the body, the skin will start to struggle with being able to detox itself in the right manner.

When you decide to go on the alkaline diet, you will find that it can help to clear up the skin. The acid is released, which frees up more room on the skin in order to detox and clear it up. This is why many people who decide to go on the alkaline diet are going to benefit throughout the entirety of their skin as well.

As you can see, simply by changing up the eating patterns that you have and making sure that you consume just foods that are considered alkaline rather than foods that are more acidic (for the most part at least), you will be able to help improve your overall health and make yourself feel so much better in the process as well! It may take some time, and you are going to need to remove some of the foods that you usually love from your diet plan, but in the long run, it can be worth it for all the great health benefits you are going to get!

Chapter 3

All about the Foods

Now that we know a bit more about the alkaline diet and all of the different parts that come with it, it is time for us to focus a bit more on some of the foods that are allowed on this diet plan. It is important to know which foods are considered alkaline and which ones are considered more acidic. Eating the wrong ones or at least too much of the wrong ones are going to bring about a bunch of illnesses and other issues in your body as well. But when you are able to focus on healthy foods, the ones that are considered alkaline, you will find that your health can improve in no time.

There are some surprises that fall on both lists, and you may be interested in seeing which foods work the best, and which ones do not when it comes to following the alkaline diet. Let's take a look at some of the eating habits that you should have when you go on this diet, which foods are considered alkaline and which ones are acidic, and even a look at what alkaline water is all about and why some people swear by its effects when they are trying to lower the acidity in their own bodies.

The Best Foods to eat that are Alkaline

While you may need to give up some of your favorite foods when you go on this diet plan, you will find that there are a ton of different foods that you get to enjoy. The first group that we need to take a look at is all the fresh produce that is encouraged to enjoy. You can consume lots of fruits and vegetables in abundance, as long as you make sure to get plenty of variety to keep your body healthy. This produce will help to provide the body with the nutrients and minerals that you need to stay healthy and can really help to detox the body and make it as healthy as possible.

All fruits and vegetables are going to be fine when you are on this diet plan so you will have a lot of variety in your diet. The next food to consider is fresh fish. All fishes are great on this kind of diet because they are not going to include some of the acid-causing nutrients that we see in red meat while providing you with the healthy fats that you need and the healthy protein. It is a great idea to try and add these into your diet at least two or three times a week, if not more. There are a lot of different options for fresh fish that you are able to choose from, so you will never get bored!

White meat options are going to be good here as well, including lots of chicken and turkey. When you aren't eating fish for one of your meals, adding these in will help you to get more protein in and to complete out your meal in an alkaline manner. These also have some added nutrients that you may not have seen with some of the other options or that are not found with fish all of the time. Add them into a sandwich or a salad or eat them on their own, just make sure that you don't try to deep fry them.

Eggs, in certain cases, are going to be fine on this diet plan. You do not want to cook them too much, or they will bring out their acid forming method possible. Eggs that are prepared lightly, such as poaching or boiling them, are the best option. Others choose to not eat the eggs at all because they are seen as slightly acidic. All of the great health benefits often outweigh the slight amount of acidity that is found in them, so these are usually seen as fine to consume on the alkaline diet.

Legumes are technically fine when you follow this plan, but you should listen to your body about them. Some people find that they have a hidden sensitivity to the legumes, which manes that they are still going to react with inflammation if they are not careful with their consumption of these. You may want to take them out of your diet for a few weeks or so, and then slowly add them back in to see whether they cause an issue or not.

Next on the list is going to be some natural nuts. You do not want to pick out any nuts that have added salt or sugar found on them because this changes things up. But regular, all-natural nuts are a good snack to add into your day, one that is going to make you feel amazing will add in the healthy fats that you need, and even more protein for the muscles.

While you do need to limit the number of whole grains, rice, and pasta to some extent, eating the whole wheat and whole grain options is the best. There are a few grains, like the processed and white grains, that you need to avoid because they are going to raise the acid level in the body, along with your insulin levels and blood sugar. But smaller amounts of the whole grain varieties will be just fine when you follow this diet.

This does not mean that you should avoid all of the grains that are out there. Whole grains are going to be full of lots of nutrients that the body should not miss out on, they can fill you up, and if you are eating the right kinds, they are going to ensure that you stay healthy and see stabilization in your blood sugars. We can all agree that these things are good and healthy for you. Stick with the whole grain pasta and rice and bread, and avoid the white bread and pastas as well as baked goods.

Spices and herbs are recommended on this plan as well. You are able to consume as many of these on this diet plan as you would like. They are a great way to add in some new flavoring and changes to your diet without having to worry about adding more acid to your body in the process. Experiment a bit with the different options that are out there and see what they are able to do with the meals that you eat.

The drinks that you choose are also important. You will find that for the most part, sticking with water is the best choice. There are some people who say that alkaline water is the best option, but any kind of regular water is just fine as well. You can also mix it up with a bit of green tea as well if you want something different.

There are so many good foods and meals that you are able to have when you go on this kind of diet plan. You just need to prepare yourself and make some adjustments to the foods that you are eating to see which ones are going to work the best for you. Sure, there may be some foods on this list that you are sad to see go, but as you look through some of the amazing recipes that we have at the end of this guidebook, you will find that there are a ton of tasty options that can make your meals as delicious as possible.

The Worst Foods that are High in Acid

It is also important to make sure that you avoid any foods that are going to be high in acid or you will ruin all of your best efforts when it comes to the alkaline diet. You are allowed to eat a few of these foods on occasion, so they don't need to be eliminated, but you must be careful not to allow them to become the main foods that you are consuming. Those need to be reserved for the alkaline foods that we talked about before. Some of the foods that you should be careful about while on this diet because they can raise the acidity level in your body will include:

1. Foods that are high in sodium. This would include any processed foods. This will constrict the blood vessels while increasing blood pressure, increasing the risk that you have for hypertension. Having salt on occasion is not a bad thing, but many meals have more than your daily amount in one serving. Learning how to limit these can help your health so much.

2. Cold cuts and other conventional meats. These are so processed that they can cause a lot of acid problems in the body.

3. Processed cereals. Cereal, on their own, is not bad, but so many have additives and preservatives that it makes them unhealthy to enjoy.

4. Caffeinated drinks and alcohol. There are some problems with these drinks due to the caffeine, the sweeteners, and the bubbles. All of these, on their own, can cause acid levels to rise in the body, and together, they make the problem worse.

5. Some wheat and oat products. You do not need to get rid of them all of the time, but you should limit your consumption a bit. Americans often fill up on these oat

and wheat products too much, and that can cause a lot of problems with acid levels. Learning how to restrict down to just a few times a day and eating the whole grain options instead is the best choice for you.

6. Milk: Eating a bit of dairy product is not a big deal. But milk and other dairy products are often going to cause more acid in the body. You should consider going with other forms of calcium like green leafy veggies, in order to get the nutrients that you need.

7. Peanuts. Some nuts are just fine and can give you the fats and protein that you need. But others, like peanuts and walnuts, are not going to be good for your body at all and should be avoided.

8. Any packaged product: This means that you really need to watch out for packaged pasta, rice, bread, and baked goods. These are not the best options for you, and it is often the best option to choose something else.

Having these food choices on occasion is not going to be that big of a deal. But for the most part, learning how to avoid them and take care of your health with more of the alkaline friendly foods, rather than the acid-friendly foods will help to keep your body healthy.

Alkaline Diet Water

Many times, we hear about the alkaline diet, and the topic of alkaline water starts to come up. There are a lot of people who will make claims about alkaline water and how it is the best option for your needs. Some believe that it is able to slow down the aging process, can help when it is time to balance your pH levels and can prevent a lot of chronic diseases that are becoming more prevalent in our modern society. But what is alkaline water and why is there a lot of hype that comes with it.

When we are talking about alkaline water, we are monitoring the levels of its pH. The pH level includes numbers that measure a substance's alkalinity and acidity based on a scale that goes from 0 to 14. For example, if a thing has a pH level of 1, it is considered very acidic. It is considered very alkaline if it reaches the pH level of 14.

Alkaline water is going to come at a higher pH level than what we see with regular drinking water. Because of this fact, there are a lot of proponents who believe that this water is the perfect addition to your diet to neutralize the acid that is found in your body. Normal drinking water is going to be neutral, which means it has a 7 as its pH level. Alkaline water is going to have a pH that is a bit higher at 8 or 9.

There is a bit more that comes with alkaline water than just the pH levels that you see. In addition to being slightly alkaline, this kind of water needs to contain minerals that are considered alkaline and an ORP or negative oxidation-reduction potential. This is referred to as the water's ability to function as an antioxidant or pro-oxidant. The more negative you are able to get the ORP value of something, the more antioxidizing it will be.

There is a bit of controversy found with alkaline water in many cases. Health professionals often worry because there isn't a lot of research out there in order to support all of the health claims that are out there. The difference in the findings of the research that has been done is related to the types of alkaline water studies.

For most people, according to the Mayo Clinic, it is best to go with regular water. There is really no scientific evidence, according to the Mayo Clinic, that will verify the claims of alkaline water's supporters. With that said, there are still some studies out there that show us how certain conditions can be assisted with the use of alkaline water.

In one study done in 2012, it was found that drinking naturally-carbonated artesian well alkaline water that had a pH level around 8.8 may help to deactivate pepsin, which is the main enzyme that is going to cause acid reflux in most people. In a second study, it was suggested that drinking alkaline water could help to control high cholesterol, diabetes, and high blood pressure.

In one study that was done more recently, there were 100 people studied, and there was a distinct difference in the blood's whole viscosity after the individuals consumed water high in pH compared to drinking regular water when they were done with a really hard work out. The viscosity is going to be a direct measurement of how efficiently the blood is able to make it through the vessels.

The viscosity is reduced by about 6.3 percent for those who consume water with high pH levels. On the other hand, the people who drink standard purified drinking water are only reduced by 3.36 percent. This means that when the participants drank the alkaline water, the blood was able to flow more efficiently, ensuring that there is an increased amount of oxygen delivered through the body.

These studies are relatively small right now, which means that we will need more information before we are able to use them to help us get the answers to whether alkaline water works or not. But for many people who decide to go on the alkaline diet, they have found that it is going to help them to reduce the amount of acidity that you are able to find in the body, so it may be worth your time to try it out at least.

This brings up the question of where you are going to be able to find this alkaline water. You are going to be able to find it online, along with many health food and grocery stores. You can also work with water ionizers also found in many large stores.

If you feel like it, you can also make it at your own home. Although the juices of both lemon and lime are considered acidic, they include some minerals that will, once digested and metabolized, create alkaline by-products. You can actually make your body more alkaline by drinking water with an added lime or lemon juice, even just a squeeze of it. Or you can add in baking soda or pH drops to make your own alkaline water.

The way that you eat during the day is going to make a big difference in how much acidity and how much alkalinity is found throughout the body. The more that you are able to limit the acidic foods, the healthier is it going to be for the whole body. It may take some time, but you will find that you can easily adjust to the many delicious alkaline foods while giving your body the best health possible in the process.

Chapter 4

The 10-Day Meal Plan

One thing that a lot of people will struggle with when they start on a new diet or eating plan is what they should eat! They may have a long list of foods that are allowed and foods that are not allowed, but knowing how to put these together and make some tasty and easy meals can be a challenge. Often, people are going to fall off the diet plan because they are bored with the food and menu choices, or they think it is too hard to find foods that they enjoy.

That is where this 10-day meal plan is going to come into play! We are going to take some of the delicious meals that are found in this guidebook and put them together to make the best meals and desserts possible for your needs! When you are ready to follow the alkaline diet, and you want to know the best meals to eat for the first ten days, make sure to use the meal plan provided to you below

Day 1:	Day 2:	Day 3:
Breakfast; Chia Parfait	Breakfast: Warm Apple Pie Cereal	Breakfast: Tofu Scramble
Lunch: Southwest Stuffed Sweet Potatoes	Lunch: Zoodles with Cream Sauce	Lunch: Rainbow Pad Thai
	Dinner: Coconut	

Dinner: Vegetable and Salmon Kebabs Dessert: Cookie Dough Bites	Curry with Vegetables Dessert: Cashew Chip Cookies	Dinner: Loaded Spaghetti Squash Dessert: Lemon Cookies
Day 4: Breakfast: Sweet Potato Parfait Lunch: Lentils and Greens Dinner: Spicy Pasta Dessert: Lemon Lime Jelly	Day 5: Breakfast: Tofu Morning Sandwich Lunch: Sesame Greens Dish Dinner: Stuffed Peppers Dessert: Strawberry Lime Bites	Day 6: Breakfast: Nutty Overnight Oats Lunch: Sweet Spinach Salad Dinner: Baba Ganoush Pasta Dessert: Coconut Chip Bites
Day 7: Breakfast: Sunnyside Breakfast Bowl Lunch: Steamed Green Bowl Dinner: Cheesy Broccoli Bowl Dessert: Sweet Potato Orange Cookies	Day 8: Breakfast: Breakfast Fruit Cups Lunch: Vegetable and Berry Salad Dinner: Green Bean and Lentil Salad Dessert: Cashew Cold Cookies	Day 9: Breakfast: Fruity Breakfast Salad Lunch: Quinoa and Carrot Bowl Dinner: Vegetable Minestrone Dessert: Pumpkin Cups

Day 10: Breakfast: Mocha Pudding Lunch: Grab and Go Wraps Dinner: Southwest Burger Dessert: Apricot Crumble		

Chapter 5

The Breakfast Recipes You Need

Chia Parfait

What's inside:
- Diced mango (.25 c.)
- Mashed raspberries (.25 c.)
- Coconut flakes (1 Tbsp.)
- Chopped cashews (2 Tbsp.)
- Nutmeg (.25 tsp.)
- Cinnamon (.25 tsp.)
- Vanilla (.5 tsp.)
- Chia seeds (3 Tbsp.)
- Almond milk (.75 c.)

How to make:
1. To start this recipe, take the cashews, nutmeg, cinnamon, vanilla, chia seeds, and almond milk.
2. Let this sit overnight in the glass jar in the fridge overnight.

3. In the morning, layer on the coconut flakes, mango, and raspberries and then serve.

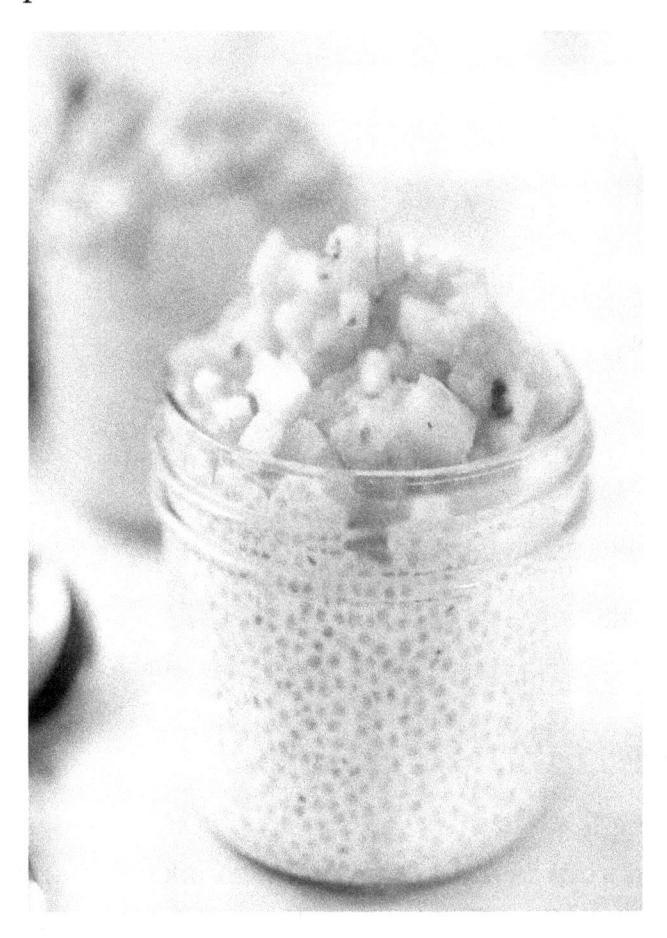

Warm Apple Pie Cereal

What's inside:

- Maple syrup (1 tsp.)
- Chopped raw almonds (.25 c.)
- Diced Granny Smith apple (1)
- Raisins (.25 c.)
- Juiced lemon (.5)
- Pinch of nutmeg
- Pinch of allspice
- Cinnamon (.5 tsp.)
- Vanilla (.25 tsp.)
- Almond milk, unsweetened (1.5 c.)
- Quinoa (.5 c.)

How to make:

1. To start, take the quinoa, almond milk, vanilla, cinnamon, allspice, nutmeg, juiced lemon, raisins, and apple into a pan and turn it on to medium heat.
2. Bring this to a gentle simmer and then reduce the heat to low. Cook until the quinoa is fluffy and the liquid is all gone.
3. Move this over to the serving bowl you want to use and then top with the maple syrup and almonds.

Tofu Scramble

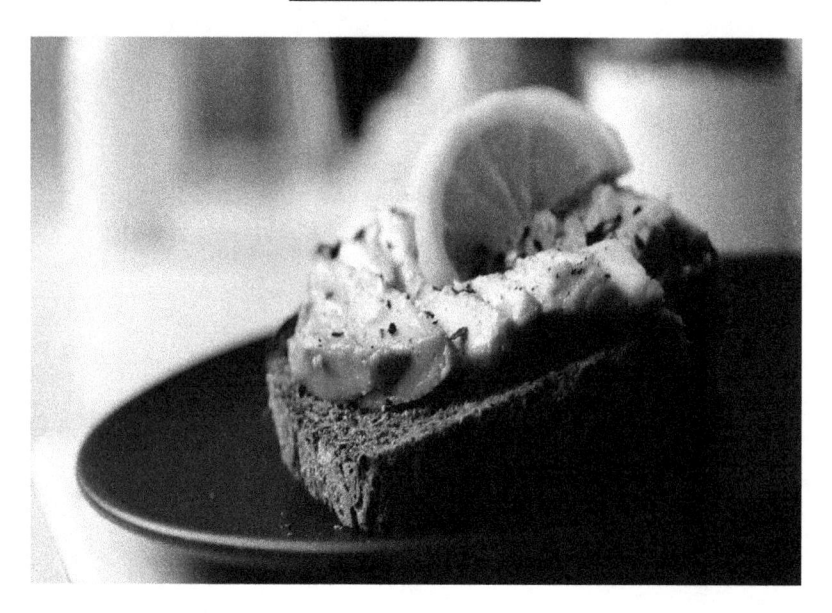

What's inside:

- Sliced avocado (1)
- Cilantro (1 Tbsp.)
- Water (3 Tbsp.)
- Pepper
- Salt
- Nutritional yeast (.5 c.)
- Turmeric (.5 tsp.)
- Cumin (.5 tsp.)
- Cubed tofu, firm (.5 block)

- Broccoli (1 c.)
- Sliced shallots (2)
- Red bell pepper (1)
- Olive oil (1 Tbsp.)

How to make:

1. To start this recipe, take some oil and add it to a skillet. Let it heat up before adding in the bell pepper, shallots, and broccoli.

2. After a few minutes of cooking this, add the tofu into this mixture, crumbling it up with a spoon. Cook for a bit longer.

3. While those ingredients are cooking, mix together the water, yeast, turmeric, pepper, cumin, salt, paprika and toss around to coat.

4. Add this to a skillet and coat well. Cook this all until you are out of liquid and then add the cilantro.

5. Move this all over to a plate, making sure to top with the prepared avocado and serve.

Sweet Potato Parfait

What's inside:

- Coconut flakes (1 Tbsp.)
- Chopped walnuts (1 Tbsp.)
- Sweet potato, remove the flesh (1)
- Cinnamon .25 tsp.)
- Nutmeg (.25 tsp.)
- Grated ginger (.5 tsp.)
- Raw honey (1 tsp.)
- Plain yogurt (1 c.)

How to make:

1. When you are ready to start, take .75 cup of the yogurt and mix it with the nutmeg, ginger, and cinnamon. Set this to the side.
2. While the cooked sweet potato is warm, mash up the potato a bit.
3. In a bowl or a jar, add in the potato on the bottom. Add in some yogurt, a few walnuts, and coconut flakes.
4. Repeat these layers until you have used up all of the ingredients.

Tofu Morning Sandwich

What's inside:

- Sliced avocado (1)
- Toasted sprouted bread (2 slices)
- Nutritional yeast (3 Tbsp.)
- Water (2 Tbsp.)
- Pepper
- Salt
- Garlic powder (1 tsp.)
- Dried oregano (1 tsp.)
- Turmeric (1 tsp.)
- Tofu (.5 block)
- Sliced shallot (1)
- Chopped broccoli (.5 c.)
- Coconut oil (1 tsp.)

How to make:

1. Bring out a big skillet and heat up your oil inside. When the oil is nice and warm, add in the shallot and broccoli. Crumble in the tofu and let it warm up.
2. While that is cooking, take out a bowl and combine together half the yeast with the water, pepper, salt, garlic, oregano, and turmeric.

3. Add this spice mixture into the broccoli and tofu mixture and then cook until the liquid has time to absorb.

4. Spoon this mixture on top of the toasted bread along with the avocado and the rest of the nutritional yeast.

Nutty Overnight Oats

What's inside:

- Hemp hearts (1 Tbsp)
- Chopped Granny Smith apple (1)
- Almond butter (2 Tbsp.)
- Salt (.25 tsp.)
- Nutmeg (1 tsp.)
- Cinnamon (1 tsp.)
- Vanilla (1 tsp.)
- Unsweetened almond milk (2 c.)
- Uncooked oats (1 c.)

How to make:

1. Take out a bowl and combine together the salt, nutmeg, cinnamon, vanilla, almond milk, and oats.

2. When this mixture is done, divide it up into two jars and shake around a bit. Place into the fridge overnight.

3. When it is time to eat this oatmeal, add in the hemp hearts, chopped apple, and almond butter to the jars before serving.

Sunnyside Breakfast Bowl

What's inside:

- Toasted pumpkin seeds (2 Tbsp.)
- Breakfast radish (1 sliced)
- Sliced avocado (1)
- Sliced scallions (2)
- Halved grape tomatoes (.5 c.)
- Salt (.5 tsp.)
- Water (3 c.)
- Yellow split peas (.75 c.)
- Sliced kale, bunch (.5)
- Minced garlic cloves (2)
- Diced shallots (2)
- Turmeric 1 tsp.)
- Coconut oil (1 Tbsp.)

How to make:

1. Take out a pan and place the coconut oil inside to heat up. When the oil is warm, you can add in the kale, garlic, shallots, and turmeric.
2. Cook these until the kale has time to wilt and then add in the split peas to cook for a bit.

3. Pour the salt and water into the pan and then bring it to a boil. Reduce the heat a bit and then let this all simmer together for a bit.

4. After ten minutes, you can divide up the mixture between a few bowls. Top this with some pumpkin seeds, radish, avocado, scallions, and tomatoes before serving.

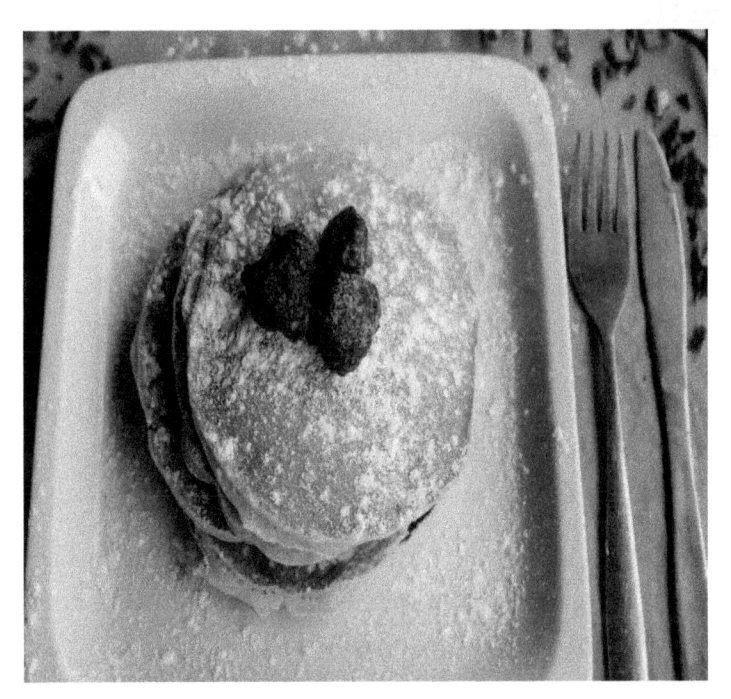

Breakfast Fruit Crepes

What's inside:

- Cacao nibs (1 Tbsp.)
- Raspberries (2 c.)
- Cashew butter (.33 c.)

- Melted ghee (2 Tbsp.)
- Water (2 c.)
- Cinnamon (.25 tsp.)
- Vanilla (.5 tsp.)
- Coconut sugar (.5 tsp.)
- Salt (.5 tsp.)
- Melted coconut oil (1 Tbsp.)
- Buckwheat flour (1 c.)
- Water (6 Tbsp.)
- Ground flax (2 Tbsp.)

How to make:

1. Take out a bowl and whisk together the water and the ground flax. Place this into the fridge to set for a bit until you see a gel form.
2. After this is done, place this mixture into the blender along with the cinnamon, vanilla, sugar, salt, coconut oil, buckwheat, and two cups of water.
3. Blend the mixture well and then set aside.
4. Add the ghee to a skillet and place on medium-low heat. Add in some of the batters to the pan, swirling it around to make a layer that is even.

5. Let this cook for a few minutes until done. And then remove from the skillet before repeating these steps. Finish up all of the batters.
6. When the crepes have a moment to cool, add in some of the cacao nibs, raspberries, and cashew butter before serving.

Fruity Breakfast Salad

What's inside:

- Raw honey (1 tsp.)
- Lime zest (1 Tbsp.)
- Unsweetened yogurt (.5 c.)
- Crushed almonds (1 Tbsp.)
- Pomegranate seeds (.25 c.)
- Sliced blood orange (1)
- Sliced persimmon fruit (1)

How to make:

1. To start this recipe, bring out a bowl and combine together the almonds, pomegranate seeds, blood orange, and persimmon.
2. Divide this mixture between two plates evenly.
3. Take out a smaller bowl and whisk together the honey, lime zest, and yogurt.

4. Top each plate with some of the yogurt mixtures before serving.

Mocha Pudding

What's inside:

- Raw cacao nibs (1 Tbsp.)
- Raspberries (.25 c.)
- Sliced banana (.5)
- Cinnamon (1 tsp.)
- Raw cacao (1 tsp)
- Brewed coffee (2 Tbsp.)
- Chia seeds (.25 c.)
- Vanilla (.5 tsp.)
- Almond milk (1 c.)

How to make:

1. To start this recipe, bring out a bowl and combine the cinnamon, cacao, coffee, chia seeds, vanilla, and almond milk.

2. Stir this together in order to combine, add a lid to the bowl, and place in the fridge overnight.

3. The next day, when you are ready to eat this dish, top it with the cacao nibs, raspberries, and banana and then serve.

Broccoli Omelet

What's inside:

- Green onions (2 Tbsp.)
- Crushed pepper (.25 tsp.)
- Turmeric (.25 tsp.)
- Dijon mustard (1 tsp.)
- Tapioca starch (3 Tbsp.)
- Nutritional yeast (3 Tbsp.)
- Unsweetened almond milk (3 Tbsp.)
- Tofu, firm (12 oz.)

The filling

- Nutritional yeast (2 Tbsp.)
- Sliced shallot (1)
- Steamed broccoli (1 c.)

How to make:

1. To start this recipe, bring out a blender and mix together the pepper, turmeric, mustard, tapioca, nutritional yeast, almond milk, and tofu.
2. Heat up a skillet until it is really hot, and then pour this batter into the skillet to cook.

3. After 7 minutes, this part will be done. Place the ingredients for the filling on one side of the omelet and then flip it over to the other side to cover.

4. Cook a bit longer before moving to a plate and garnishing with green onions to enjoy.

<u>Tofu and Kale Tacos</u>

What's inside:

- Sliced avocado (1)
- Chopped cilantro (1 Tbsp.)
- Greed onions, sliced (1 Tbsp.)
- Warmed corn tortillas (4)
- Halved cherry tomatoes (5)
- Sliced kale (1 c.)
- Coconut aminos (1 Tbsp.)
- Turmeric (.25 tsp.)
- Onion powder (1 tsp.)
- Nutritional yeast (2 Tbsp.)
- Tofu (7 oz.)
- Coconut oil (1 Tbsp.)

How to use:

1. To start this recipe, bring out a skillet and heat up the coconut oil inside. When the oil is warm, add in the coconut aminos, turmeric, onion powder, and nutritional yeast with the tofu.
2. After cooking for 5 minutes, you can add in the cherry tomatoes and the kale and cook for a bit longer.
3. Take this kale and tofu mixture off the stove and divide up among the four corn tortillas.
4. Top this with the avocado, cilantro, and green onions before serving.

Savory Breakfast Bowl

What's inside:

- Sliced green onion (1 Tbsp.)
- Cooked lentils (.33 c.)
- Red chili flakes (.25 tsp.)
- Turmeric (.5 tsp.)
- Lemon zest (1 tsp.)
- Nutritional yeast (1 Tbsp.)
- Spinach (1 c.)
- Pepper (.25 tsp.)
- Salt (.25 tsp.)
- Water (.5 c.)

- Unsweetened almond milk (.5 c.)
- Rolled oats (.5 c.)

How to make:

1. Take out a pan and heat up the pepper, salt, water, almond milk, and oats inside.
2. Let these reach a boil before reducing the heat to a simmer to cook for a bit. After five to ten minutes, the liquid should be mostly absorbed.
3. When this happens, stir in the lentils, chili flakes, turmeric, lemon zest, nutritional yeast, and spinach.
4. Take off the stove and then garnish with some green onions before you serve.

Almond Butter and Jelly Overnight Oats

What's inside:

- Sliced raspberries (4)
- Sliced almonds (1 Tbsp.)
- Almond butter (1 Tbsp.)
- Chia seeds (1 tsp.)
- Vanilla (.5 tsp.)
- Almond milk (.75 c.)
- Rolled oats (.5 c.)

For the jam

- Chia seeds (1 Tbsp.)
- Honey (1 tsp.)
- Mashed raspberries (.25 c.)

How to make:

1. To start this recipe, take .25 cup of mashed raspberries and combine with the tablespoon of the chia seeds with the honey.
2. Combine these ingredients together well and then put into the fridge to set for a bit.
3. After ten minutes, add in a tablespoon of this raspberry mixture with the chia seeds, vanilla, almond milk, and oats into a jar. Mix the ingredients together well.
4. Cover the jar and let it set in the fridge for 8 hours or more.
5. When it is time to serve the next day, add in the almond butter, the rest of the raspberries, and the almonds before serving.

Chapter 6

Easy Smoothie Recipes

Tropical Smoothie

What's inside:
- Coconut water (.5 c.)
- Chopped cilantro (.5 c.)
- Steamed cauliflower florets (.5 c.)
- Limes juiced (2)
- Diced watermelon (1 c.)
- Diced pineapple (1 c.)

How to make:
1. Add all of your ingredients into a blender and blend until nice and smooth.
2. Divide this smoothie between two cups before serving.

Ginger Smoothie

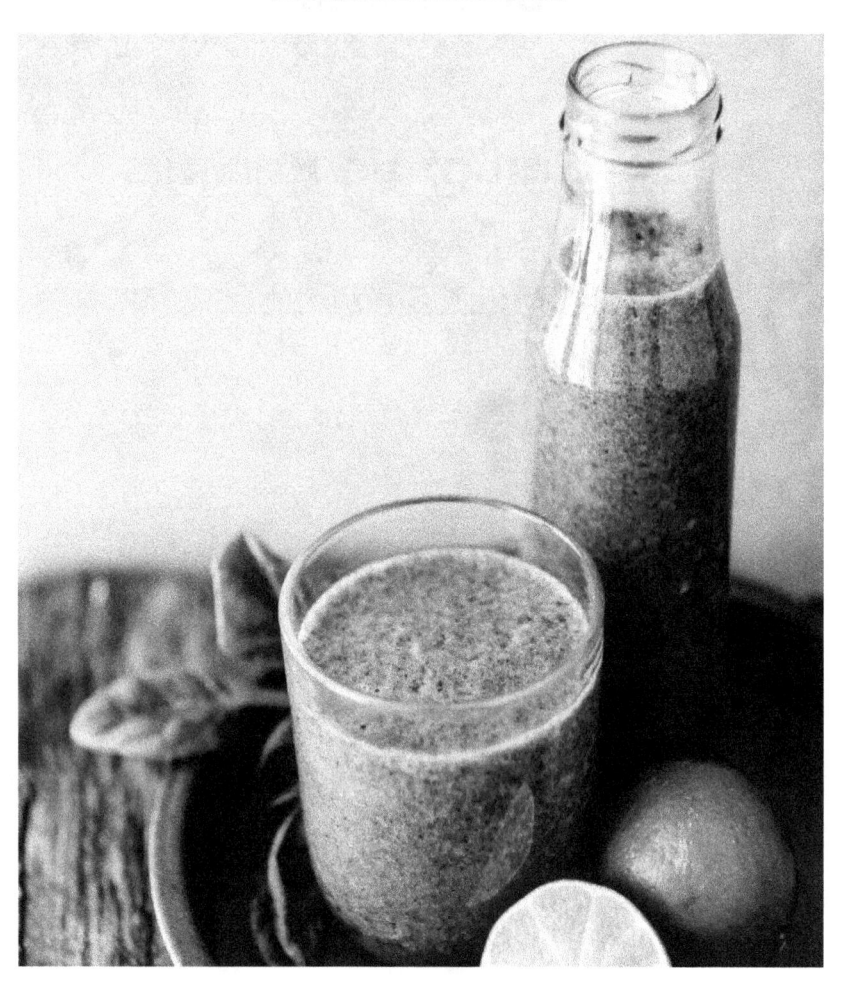

What's inside:

- Chia seeds (2 tsp.)
- Water (1 c.)
- Chopped apple (1)

- Spinach (2 c.)
- Ginger, sliced (2-inch piece)
- Juiced lime (1)
- Juiced lemon (1)
- Chopped cucumbers (2)

How to make;

1. Bring out your blender and add in all of the ingredients above except for the chia seeds.
2. Blend those ingredients together well until they are smooth. Pour the drink into two glasses.
3. Stir in the chia seeds before serving.

Vegetable Smoothie

What's inside:

- Turmeric (1-inch piece)
- Ginger (1-inch piece)
- Parsley (.5 c.)
- Lemon (.5)
- Kale (1 c.)
- Green cabbage (.25 head)
- Cucumber (1)
- Carrots (2)

How to make:

1. Take out a blender and add in all of the ingredients above.
2. When these are well combined, pour into two glasses before serving.

Lime and Coconut Smoothie

What's inside:

- Lime zest (.5 tsp.)
- Ice cubes (4)
- Frozen banana (1)
- Peeled lime (1)
- Coconut oil (1 Tbsp.)
- Coconut milk (.5 c.)
- Coconut water (.5 c.)
- Coconut meat (4 oz.)

How to make:

1. Take out a blender and place all of your ingredients besides the lime zest inside.
2. Blend the ingredients on a high setting until they are fully combined.
3. Pour into two glasses and garnish with the lime zest before serving.

Berry Blast Smoothie

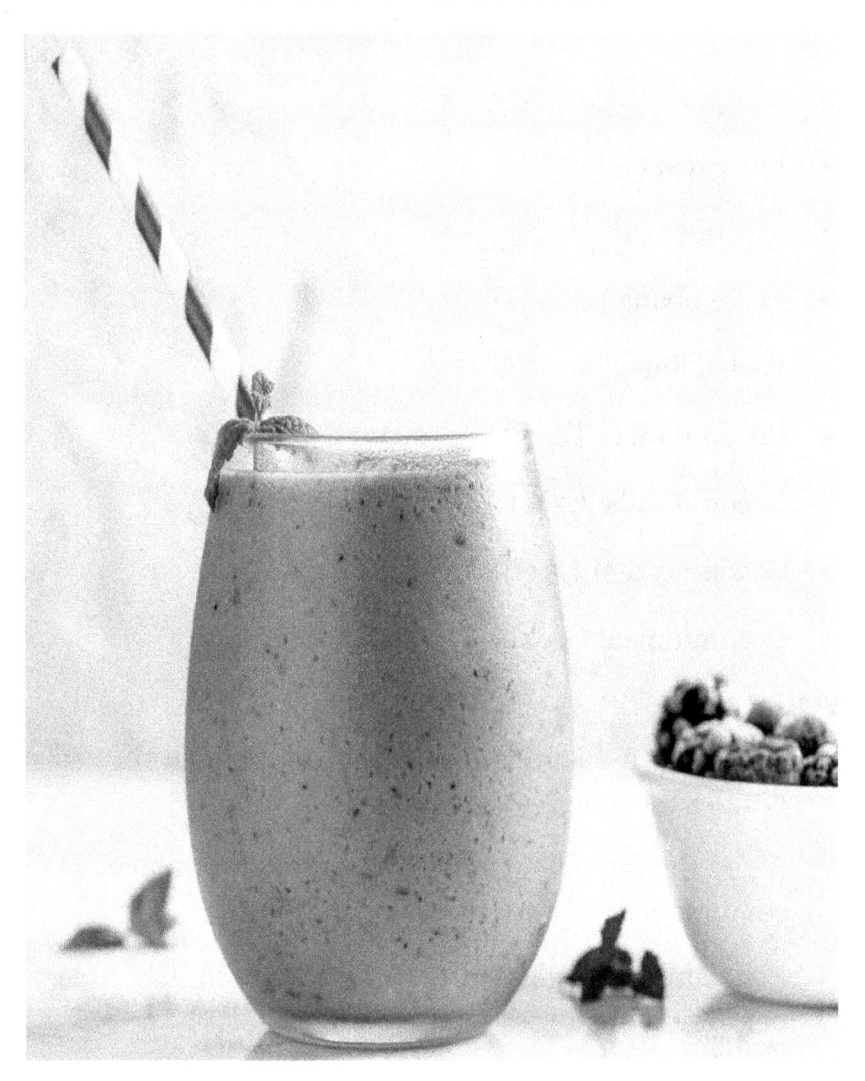

What's inside:

- Hemp hearts (1 Tbsp.)
- Chia seeds (1 Tbsp.)

- Almond milk (1 c.)
- Coconut oil (1 Tbsp.)
- Ground flaxseed (1 Tbsp.)
- Raw cashew butter (1 Tbsp.)
- Raspberries (.25 c.)
- Blueberries (.25 c.)
- Spinach (1 c.)

How to make:

1. To start this recipe, bring out the blender and add in all of your previous ingredients besides the hemp hearts and the chia seeds.

2. Place the lid on top of the blender and blend it all together to make it nice and smooth.

3. Pour the mixture into a few cups and then stir in the hemp hearts and the chia seeds before serving.

Minty Morning Shake

What's inside:

- Mint leaves (2)
- Cacao nibs (1 tsp.)
- Ice cubes (8)
- Peppermint extract (.25 tsp.)
- Salt (.25 tsp.)
- Vanilla (1 tsp.)
- Pitted dates (2)
- Frozen bananas (2)
- Mint leaves (.5 c.)
- Avocado (.5)
- Spinach (1 c.)
- Canned coconut milk (.25 c.)
- Unsweetened coconut milk (.75 c.)

How to make:

1. Take out your blender and add in the rest of the ingredients except the mint leaves and cacao nibs into the blender.
2. Blend this until smooth and then pour into two cups.

3. Garnish with the mint leaves and cacao nibs before serving.

Fruit and Green Tea Smoothie

What's inside:

- Ice cubes (3)
- Matcha green tea powder (2 tsp.)
- Juiced lime (1)
- Almond milk (1 c.)
- Peeled frozen banana (1)
- Diced pineapple (.25 c.)
- Raspberries (.5 c.)
- Chopped mangoes (2)

How to make:

1. Bring out the blender and add in all of the ingredients.
2. Blend these together until they are nice and smooth.
3. Pour the fruit and green tea mixture into two glasses and then serve.

Apple Pie Smoothie

What's inside:

- Salt (.25 tsp.)
- Vanilla (.5 tsp.)
- Nutmeg (.5 tsp.)
- Cinnamon (1 tsp.)
- Pitted and soaked dates (3)
- Almond milk (1.5 c.)
- Frozen banana (.5)
- Chopped red apple (1)

How to make:

1. Bring out a blender and add all of your ingredients from above inside.
2. Blend these together well until they are nice and smooth.
3. Pour into two glasses before serving.

Detox Juice

What's inside:

- Ginger (1.5-inch piece)
- Peeled lemon (1)
- Apple (1)
- Peeled carrot (1)
- Peeled beets (2)

How to make:

1. Add all of the above ingredients int a juicer or a blender.
2. Place the lid on top and blend the ingredients together until nice and smooth.
3. When this is done, pour into one glass before serving.

Fruity Lemonade

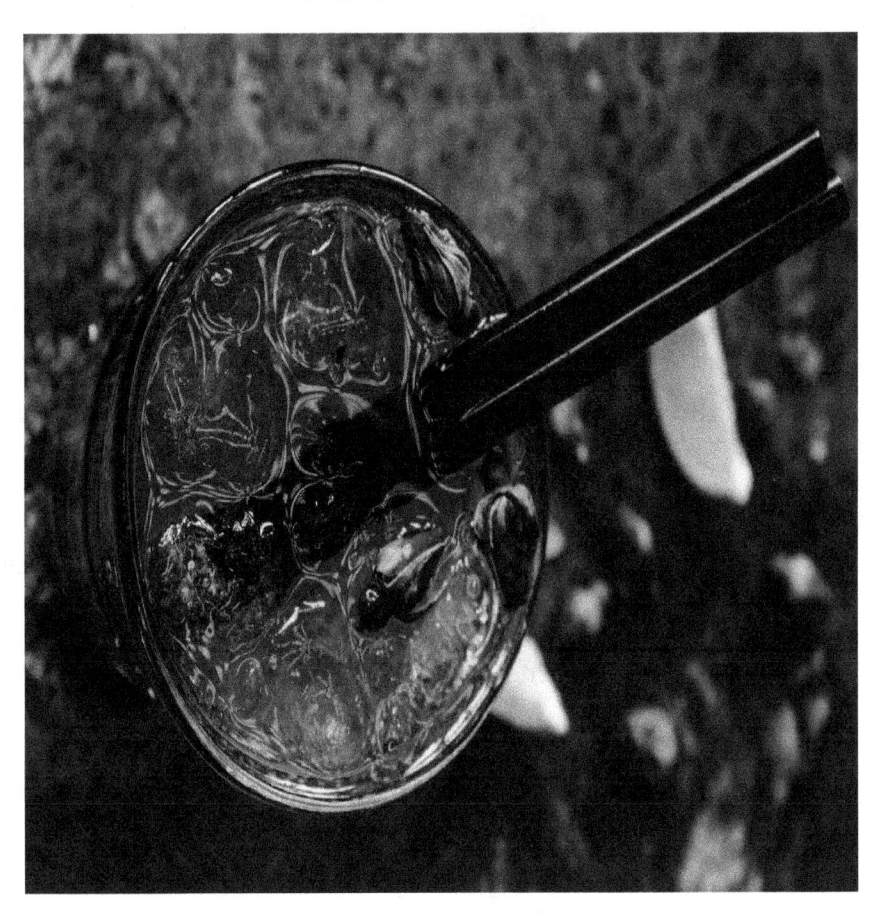

What's inside:

- Ice cubes (5)
- Raw honey (1 tsp.)
- Mint (.5 c.)
- Cubed watermelon (1 c.)

- Hulled strawberries (1 c.)
- Water (1.5 c.)
- Apple (1)
- Lemons (3)

How to make:

1. Use your juicer to juice the lemons and set this juice to the side.
2. Juice the apples in your juicer as well and add this juice in with the lemon juice inside of the blender.
3. Inside the blender, add in the ice cubes, honey, mint, watermelon, strawberries, and water. Blend these together until smooth.
4. Pour the mixture into two serving glasses and then enjoy.

Chapter 7

Lunch Recipes

Southwest Stuffed Sweet Potatoes

What's inside:

- Sliced avocado (1)
- Pinch of cumin
- Pinch of dried red chili flakes
- Spinach (3 c.)
- Sliced shallot (1)
- Black beans (.5 c.)
- Coconut oil (2 Tbsp.)
- Sweet potatoes

The dressing

- Pepper and salt
- Minced cilantro (1 handful)
- Cumin (1 tsp.)
- Juiced lime (1)

- Olive oil (3 Tbsp.)

How to make:

1. Turn on the oven and give it time to heat up to 400 degrees. Clean the sweet potatoes and pierce a few times with a fork.
2. Add some parchment paper to a baking tray and set the sweet potatoes on top. Add to the oven to bake.
3. After 50 minutes, the potatoes should be soft. Take them out of the oven and give them time to cool.
4. In the meantime, take out a skillet and add in the coconut oil along with the black beans and the shallot.
5. Cook these for a few minutes before adding in the cumin, chili flakes, and spinach, stirring around to mix well.
6. Finally, take out a small bowl and whisk the ingredients for the dressing together well.
7. Slice the sweet potatoes down the middle before stuffing with the mixture of black beans that you made.
8. Top with some of the slices of avocado along with some of the dressing drizzled on them before serving.

Zoodles with Cream Sauce

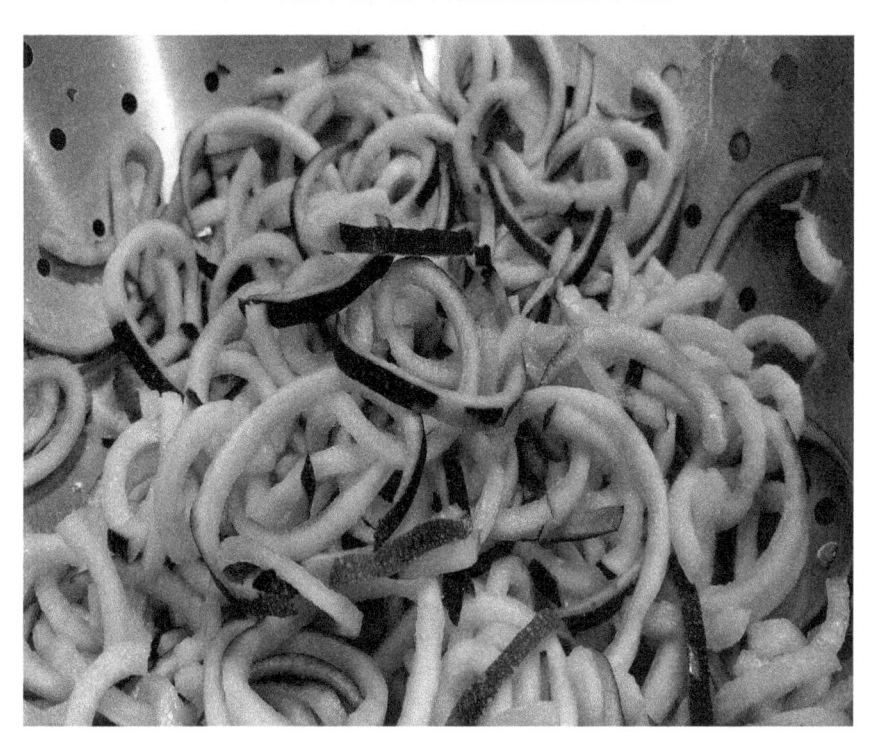

What's inside:

- Toasted pepitas (2 Tbsp.)
- Pepper (.5 tsp.)
- Salt (1 tsp.)
- Minced cilantro (2 Tbsp.)
- Water (1 Tbsp.)
- Juiced lemon (.5)
- Olive oil (2 Tbsp.)

- Pitted avocado (1)
- Spiralized zucchini (1)
- Coconut oil (1 Tbsp.)

How to make:

1. Add some coconut oil to melt on a skillet before adding in the zucchini noodles. Cook for 5 minutes before turning the heat off.
2. Take out a blender and combine together the pepper, salt, a tablespoon of cilantro, water, lemon juice, oil, and avocado. Mix well and cook to make creamy.
3. Add the sauce to the skillet with your noodles and toss to combine. Move over to a serving bowl and top with the rest of the cilantro and the toasted pepitas before serving.

Rainbow Pad Thai

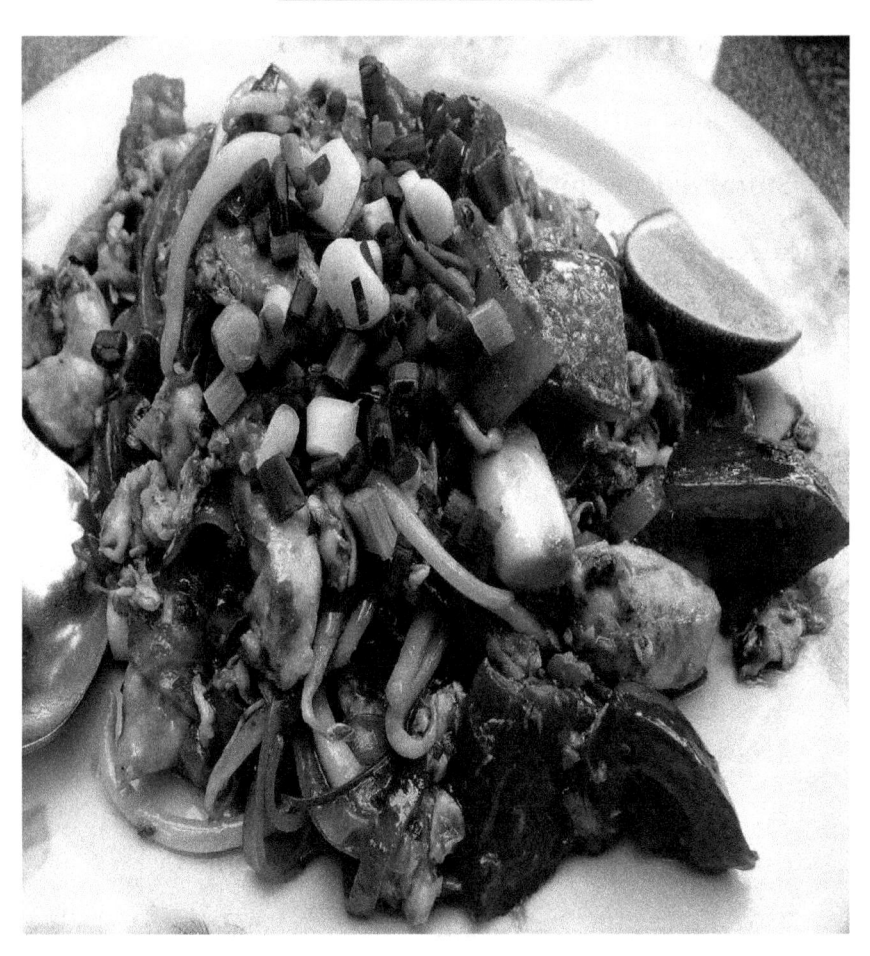

What's inside:

- Diced avocado (1)
- Chopped cilantro (1 c.)
- Shredded daikon radish (1 c.)
- Chopped broccoli (1 c.)

- Shredded red cabbage (1 c.)
- Sliced scallions (3)
- Shredded carrots (2)
- Spiralized zucchini (3)

For the dressing

- Minced ginger (1 tsp.)
- Minced garlic clove (1)
- Sesame oil (1 tsp.)
- Tahini (.25 c.)
- Juiced lime (1)

How to make:

1. Add the ingredients for the Pad Thai, except for the avocado, into a big bowl and toss around.
2. Whisk together all of the ingredients that you have for the dressing until they are creamy and combined.
3. Top the vegetables with the diced avocado and drizzle the dressing on top before serving.

Lentils and Greens

What's inside:

- Avocado (1)
- Crushed almonds (1 tsp.)
- Crushed black pepper (1 tsp.)
- Salt (1 tsp.)
- Arugula (1 c.)
- Brown or green lentils (.5 c.)
- Cooked wild rice (1 c.)
- Juiced lemon (.5)
- Diced carrot (1)
- Broccoli florets (.5 c.)
- Sliced pak choi (.5 c.)
- Vegetable broth (.25 c.)

How to make:

1. Add the vegetable broth to a skillet on medium heat. Give it some time to start simmering before adding in the lemon juice, carrot, broccoli, and pak choi.
2. After 5 minutes, turn the heat off the stove and stir in the almonds, pepper, salt, arugula, lentils, and wild rice.
3. Move this mixture over to plates and top with some avocado slices before serving.

Sesame Greens Dish

What's inside:

- Sesame seeds (1 tsp.)
- Juiced lemon (.5)
- Tamari sauce (2 Tbsp.)
- Minced garlic clove (1)
- Diced red bell pepper (.5 c.)
- Finely chopped broccoli florets (2 c.)
- Cubed tofu (8 oz.)
- Olive oil (2 Tbsp.)
- Sesame oil, toasted (1.5 Tbsp.)

How to make:

1. Heat up half a tablespoon of sesame oil and a tablespoon of olive oil in a pan. Add in the tofu and let it cook for a bit.
2. After ten minutes, take the tofu out and add in a bit more of the two oils.
3. Stir in the garlic, red bell pepper, and broccoli until they have time to soften a bit. Add in the tofu and stir in the lemon juice and the soy sauce as well.
4. Top this dish with some sesame seeds before serving.

Sweet Spinach Salad

What's inside:

- Crushed black pepper (1 tsp.)
- Salt (1 tsp.)
- Nutmeg (1 tsp.)
- Cinnamon (1 tsp.)
- Chopped spinach (4 c.)
- Chopped parsley (2 Tbsp.)
- Chopped walnuts (.25 c.)
- Raisins (.25 c.)
- Sliced apple (.5 c.)
- Yogurt (.5 c.)
- Lime juice (1 tbsp.)
- Shredded carrots (.75 c.)

How to make:

1. To start this recipe, bring out a big bowl and combine all of the ingredients together.
2. Add the bowl to the fridge to chill for about ten minutes before serving.

Steamed Green Bowl

What's inside:

- Chopped cilantro (2 Tbsp.)
- Salt (1 tsp.)
- Sliced green onions (2)
- Ground cashews (1 c.)
- Coconut milk (2 c.)
- Green peas (.5 c.)
- Sliced zucchini (1)
- Broccoli head (1)
- Grated ginger (1-inch piece)
- Turmeric (1 tsp.)
- Minced garlic clove (1)
- Sliced onion (1)
- Coconut oil (1 Tbsp.)

How to make:

1. Heat up some coconut oil in a pan and when it is warm, add in the ginger, turmeric, garlic, and onion.
2. After five minutes of cooking, add in the coconut milk, peas, zucchini, and broccoli to this mixture.

3. Let the ingredients come to a boil before reducing the heat down and simmering this for a bit.

4. After another 15 minutes, stir in the cilantro, salt, green onions, and cashews before serving.

Vegetable and Berry Salad

What's inside:

- Raspberries (.5 c.)
- Sliced tangerine (.5)
- Alfalfa sprouts (1 c.)
- Shredded red cabbage (.5 head)
- Juiced lemon 1)
- Olive oil (3 Tbsp.)
- Diced cucumber (1)
- Avocado (1)
- Sliced shallot (1)
- Sliced kale (4 leaves)
- Chopped parsley (1 Tbsp.)
- Sliced red bell pepper (.5)
- Shredded carrot (1)
- Crushed almonds (1 Tbsp.)
- Pumpkin seeds (2 Tbsp.)

How to make:

1. Take out a large bowl and add in all of the ingredients to it.
2. Toss well to combine before topping the fruits and vegetables with some lemon juice and some oil.
3. Serve this right away.

Quinoa and Carrot Bowl

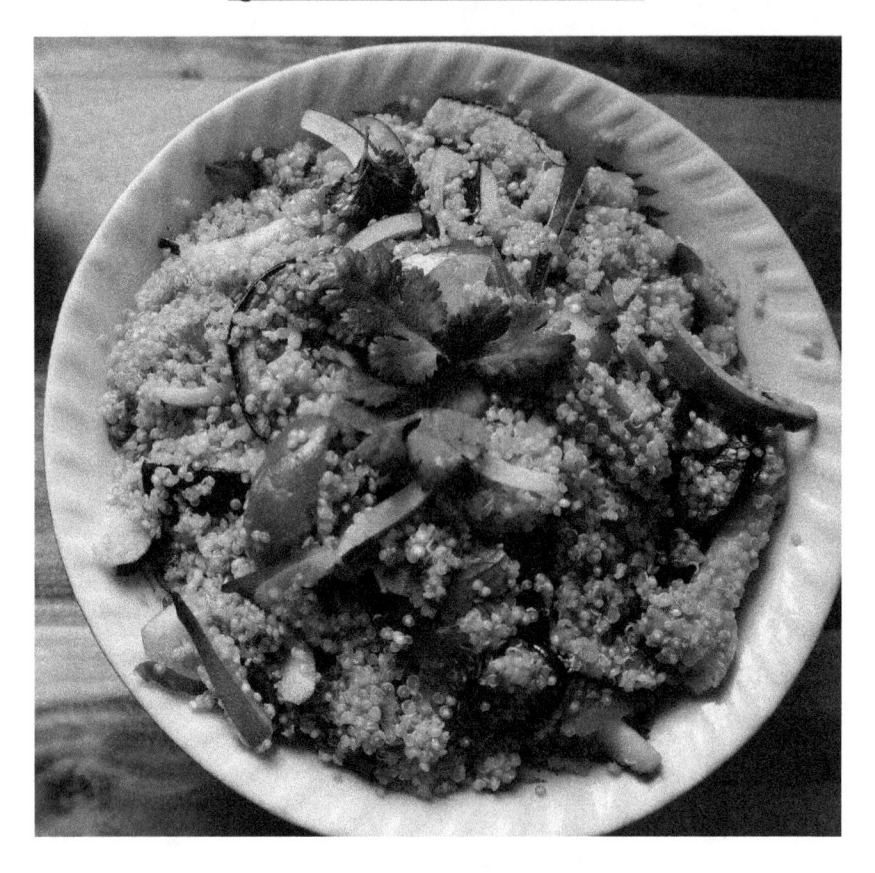

What's inside:

- Sliced green onions (2 Tbsp.)
- Black sesame seeds (2 Tbsp.)
- Salt (.25 tsp.)
- Chopped parsley (3 Tbsp.)
- Juiced lemon (.5)
- Cooked quinoa (2 c.)
- Sliced fennel bulb (1)
- Carrots, chopped (1 bunch)
- Olive oil (1 Tbsp.)
- Miso (1 Tbsp.)
- Water (1 c.)

How to make:

1. Whisk together the miso and the water in a bowl. Then take out a skillet and heat up some oil inside.
2. When the oil is warm, add in the fennel bulb and carrots and cook for a few minutes, flipping over when three minutes have passed.
3. Add the water and miso mixture to the pan and reduce the heat down to a low. Cook with the lid on for a bit. This will take 20 minutes.
4. While this mixture is cooking, combine together the quinoa with the parsley, lemon juice, and salt in a bowl.

5. When the carrots are done, add that mixture over the quinoa. Sprinkle on the green onions and sesame seeds before serving.

Grab and Go Wraps

What's inside:

- Julienned carrot (1)
- Red bell pepper (.5)
- Collard greens (4)
- Salt (.25 tsp.)
- Diced jalapeno pepper (.5)
- Diced shallot (1)
- Chopped cilantro leaves (.25 c.)
- Juiced lime (1)
- Avocado (1)
- Steamed green peas (1 c.)

How to make:

1. Take out your blender or your food processor and combine together the salt, jalapeno, shallot, cilantro, lime, avocado, and peas. The process to combine, but allow for a bit of texture to still be there.
2. Lay out the collard greens on the counter and then spread out your pea and avocado mixture to the top.
3. Add in the strips of carrots and bell peppers before rolling the collard greens up and securing with a toothpick.
4. Repeat with all of the ingredients before serving.

Nutty Tacos

What's inside:

- Chopped cilantro (1 Tbsp.)
- Nutritional yeast (2 Tbsp.)
- Lettuce leaves, romaine (6)
- Cooked red quinoa (.25 c.)
- Salt (.25 tsp.)
- Tamari (1 tsp.)
- Coconut aminos (1 tsp.)
- Smoked paprika (.25 tsp.)
- Onion powder (.25 tsp.)
- Garlic powder (.25 tsp.)
- Chili powder (.25 tsp.)
- Ground coriander (1 tsp.)
- Ground cumin (1 tsp.)
- Olive oil (2 Tbsp.)
- Chopped sun-dried tomatoes (.25 c.)
- Slivered raw almonds (.25 c.)
- Walnuts (.5 c.)

How to make:

1. To begin with this recipe, add the almonds and walnuts in the food processor and pulse together until chopped.

2. Add in the tomatoes and pulse together a few times until you get a nice crumbly mixture.

3. From here, add in the salt, tamari, coconut aminos, paprika, onion, garlic, chili, coriander, cumin, and olive oil. Pulse a few more times to get fully combined.

4. Add the tomato and nut mixture into a bowl and combine together with the quinoa.

5. Divide this mixture between the leaves of romaine lettuce and top with the cilantro and nutritional yeast before serving.

Tex-Mex Bowl

What's inside:
- Nutritional yeast (2 Tbsp.)
- Cilantro (2 Tbsp.)
- Sliced avocado (1)
- Salt (.25 tsp.)
- Olive oil (.25 c.)
- Apple cider vinegar (.25 c.)
- Juiced and zested lime (1)
- Juiced and zest lemon (1)
- Juiced oranges (2)
- Minced garlic cloves (2)
- Sliced red onion (1)
- Sliced bell peppers

For the brown rice
- Back beans (.5 c.)
- Garlic powder (.5 tsp.)
- Cayenne pepper (.5 tsp.)
- Paprika (1 tsp.)
- Salt (1 tsp.)

- Garlic powder (1.5 tsp.)
- Chili powder (2 tsp.)
- Cooked brown rice (1 c.)

Salsa

- Juice from one lime
- Salt (.25 tsp.)
- Diced cilantro (.25 c.)
- Diced red onion (.5)
- Diced tomatoes (2)

How to make:

1. Take out a big bowl and combine together the salt, olive oil, vinegar, lime zest and juice, lemon zest and juice, garlic, red onion, and the bell pepper.
2. Cover and let this set for about five hours to marinate a bit. While the peppers marinate a bit in the fridge, it is time to work on the salsa.
3. To make the salsa, add all of the ingredients in a small bowl and stir well to combine. Cover up the bowl and then place in the fridge.
4. In a medium bowl, add in all of the ingredients for the brown rice. Toss these together well and set to the side.
5. Heat up your skillet and add in the bell peppers with a bit of the marinade. Cook for a bit until the onion and bell peppers are soft.

6. Add the rice to some serving bowls and top with the bell peppers and onion mixture, the salsa, and the avocado. Top with the nutritional yeast and cilantro before serving.

Avocado Soup and Salmon

What's inside:
- Cilantro (2 Tbsp.)
- Crushed pepper (1 tsp.)
- Olive oil (1 tsp.)
- Flaked salmon (1 can)
- Salt (.25 tsp.)
- Cumin (.25 tsp.)
- Vegetable broth (1.5 c.)
- Full fat coconut cream (2 Tbsp.)
- Lemon juice (4 Tbsp.)
- Sliced green onion (1 Tbsp.)
- Chopped shallot (1)
- Pitted avocados (3)

How to make:
1. Bring out a blender and combine together the salt, cumin, vegetable broth, coconut cream, two tablespoons of lemon juice, green onion, shallot, and avocado.

2. Blend this together until smooth and then chill in the fridge for an hour.

3. In the meantime, bring out a bowl and combine a tablespoon of the cilantro, two tablespoons of lemon juice, the pepper, olive oil, and salmon together.

4. Add the chilled avocado soup in the bowls and top each with the salmon along with the rest of the cilantro. Serve right away.

Asian Pumpkin Salad

What's inside:

- Diced avocado (.5)

- Pomegranate seeds (.25 c.)

- Lemon juice (1 Tbsp.)

- Sliced kale (4 c.)

- Olive oil (1.5 Tbsp.)

- Cubed pumpkin (2 c.)

- Salt (.5 tsp.)

- Red chili flakes (.25 tsp.)

- Ground mustard (.25 tsp.)

- Ground garlic (.25 tsp.)

- Ground cloves (.25 tsp.)

- Black sesame seeds (1 Tbsp.)

- White sesame seeds (1 Tbsp.)

How to make:

1. Turn on the oven and give it time to heat up to 400 degrees. Prepare a baking tray with some parchment paper.

2. Using a large plate, combine both the black and white sesame seeds with the salt, chili flakes, mustard, garlic, and cloves.

3. Drizzle the pumpkin with a bit of olive oil and then roll each cube into the sesame seed mixture, pressing down a bit to coat.

4. Add the pumpkin to the baking tray and place into the oven. It will take half an hour to cook.

5. While the pumpkin is cooking, add the kale to a big bowl and drizzle on the salt, lemon juice, and the rest of the olive oil. Massage the mixture into the kale and then set aside.

6. When the pumpkin is done, add it on top of the kale and garnish with the avocado and pomegranate seeds before serving.

Sweet Potato Wraps

What's inside:

- Avocado (1)
- Alfalfa sprouts (1 c.)
- Sliced red onion (.5)
- Spinach (1 c.)
- Cooked quinoa (.5 c.)
- Collard greens (4)

Sweet potato hummus

- Crushed black pepper (.25 tsp.)
- Salt (.25 tsp.)
- Cinnamon powder (.25 tsp.)
- Chili powder (.25 tsp.)
- Garlic clove (1)
- Juiced lemon (.5)
- Olive oil (.25 c.)
- Tahini (.33 c.)
- Cubed sweet potato (1)

How to make:

1. Take the sweet potatoes and add them to a pan. Cover with the water and bring to a boil. When it reaches a boil, reduce the heat and let it cook for a bit to make the potatoes tender.

2. When these are done, drain out the water and add to the food processor along with the pepper, salt, cinnamon, chili powder, garlic, lemon juice, olive oil, and tahini. Process until smooth.

3. Lay out each of the collard greens and then spread the sweet potato hummus on each one.

4. Top this with the avocado, sprouts, onion, spinach, and quinoa. Roll these up and secure with toothpicks. Repeat until the greens and filling are gone.

Spicy Cabbage Bowl

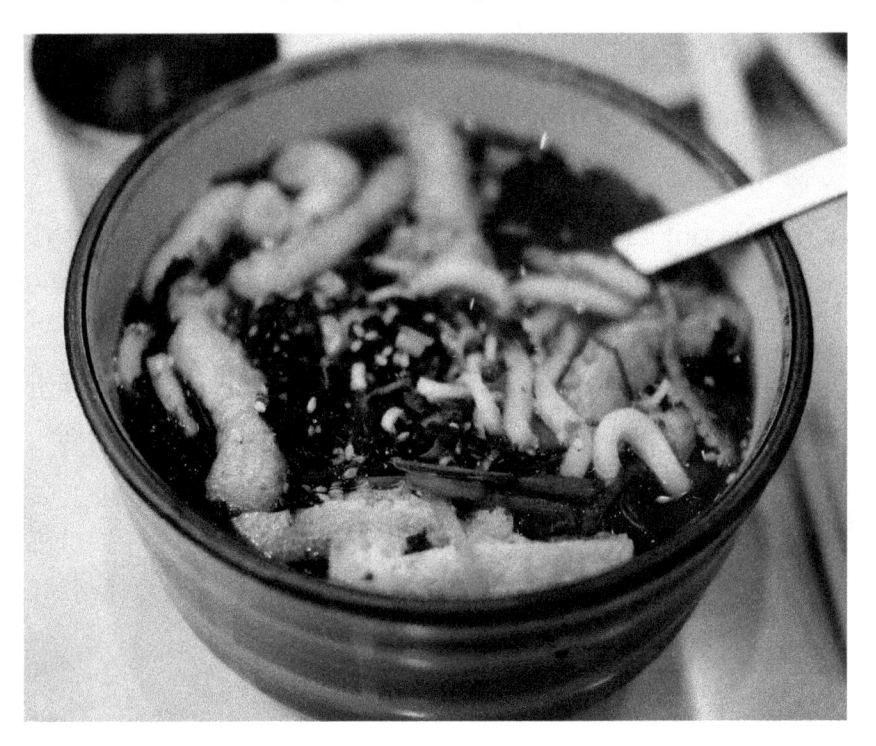

What's inside:

- Sesame seeds (1 Tbsp.)
- Green onion (.25 c.)
- Kale (2 c.)
- Coconut aminos (1 tsp.)
- Tamari (2 tsp.)
- Chopped cabbage kimchi (1 c.)
- Cooked brown rice (1 c.)

- Minced garlic (1 tsp.)
- Grated ginger (.5 tsp.)
- Sesame oil (2 tsp.)

How to make:

1. Bring out a skillet and heat up the sesame oil inside. When the oil is hot, add in the coconut aminos, tamari, kimchi, brown rice, garlic, and ginger together.
2. After five minutes of these ingredients cooking together, add in the green onions and kale and toss to combine.
3. Cook for a bit longer. Then you can garnish the dish with some sesame seeds before serving.

Citrus and Fennel Salad

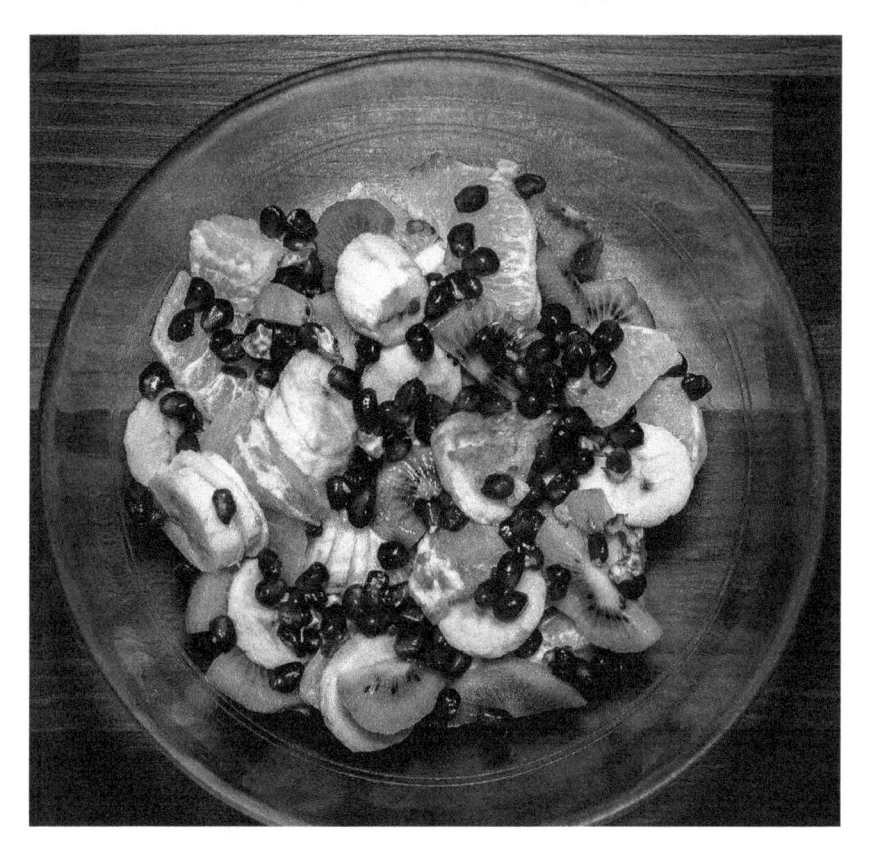

What's inside:

- Diced avocado (.5)
- Pomegranate seeds (2 Tbsp.)
- Pepper (.5 tsp.)
- Salt (.25 tsp.)
- Olive oil (.25 c.)

- Orange juice (2 Tbsp.)
- Lemon juice (2 Tbsp.)
- Chopped mint (1 Tbsp.)
- Chopped parsley (.5 c.)
- Sliced fennel bulbs (2)
- Segmented red grapefruit (.5)
- Segmented orange (1)

How to make:

1. To start this recipe, bring out a big bowl and combine together the parsley, mint, fennel slices, grapefruit segments, and orange segments. Toss to combine.
2. In another bowl, whisk together the pepper, salt, olive oil, orange juice, and lemon juice.
3. When that is combined, pour it over the fennel and citrus mixture in the big bowl, tossing around to coat.
4. Move the whole thing over to a plate and garnish with the avocado and the pomegranate seeds. Serve right away.

Chapter 8

Dinner Recipes to Bring the Family Together

Vegetable and Salmon Kebabs

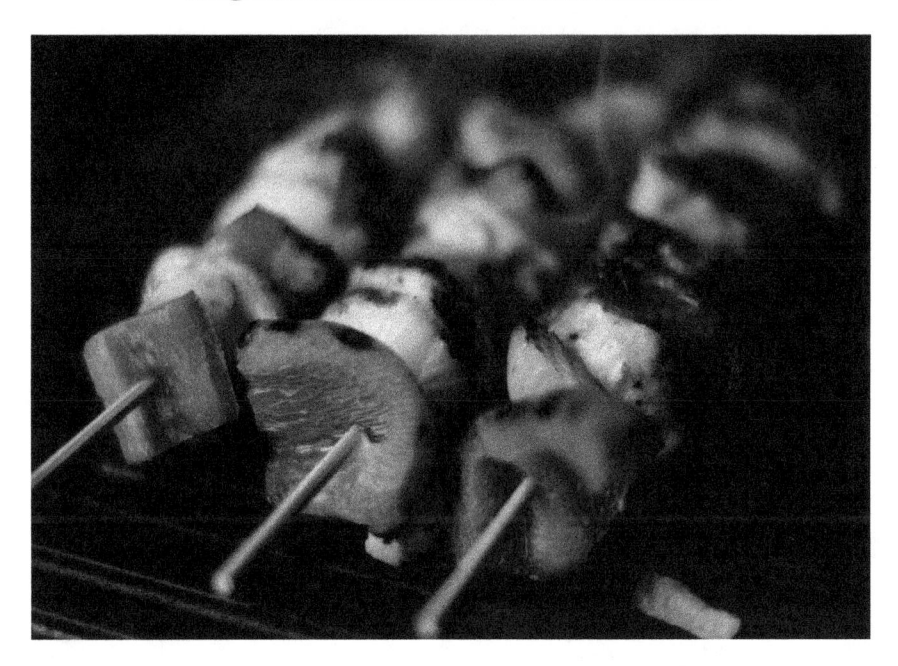

What's inside:

- 4 wooden skewers
- Pepper (.25 tsp.)

- Salt (.5 tsp.)
- Minced garlic cloves (1)
- Olive oil (1 Tbsp.)
- Quartered sweet onion (.5)
- Sliced yellow pepper (1)
- Cherry tomatoes (12)
- Chopped zucchini (1)
- Salmon (6 oz.)

For the pest sauce

- Pepper (.5 tsp.)
- Salt (1 tsp.)
- Olive oil (.25 c.)
- Pumpkin seeds (.25 c.)
- Basil leaves (.5 c.)
- Minced garlic clove (1)
- Spinach (1 c.)
- Juiced lemon (1)

How to make:

1. Take out the skewers and thread the vegetables and salmon on them in the pattern that you want.

2. Add these to a baking tray and then brush on the pepper, garlic, salt, and olive oil.

3. Turn on the oven and give it time to heat up to 400 degrees. Add the skewers into the oven and bake for a bit.

4. After 20 minutes, see if the fish is cooked through and then set to the side to cool down.

5. Bring out your blender and place all of the ingredients for the pesto sauce inside. Add in more oil if it is needed.

6. Drizzle the pesto sauce over your salmon skewers before serving.

Coconut Curry with Vegetables

What's inside:

- Chopped cilantro (3 Tbsp.)
- Curry powder (2 tsp.)
- Salt (1 tsp.)
- Water (.33 c.)
- Coconut milk (1 c.)
- Diced tomato (1)
- Firm tofu, sliced (8 oz.)
- Green beans (.25 lb.)
- Cubed eggplant (.5 c.)
- Yellow bell pepper sliced (1)
- Cubed zucchini (2)
- Diced yellow onion (.5)
- Coconut oil (2 Tbsp.)

How to make:

1. Bring out a skillet and heat up the coconut oil on it. After the oil is warm, add in the beans, eggplant, bell pepper, zucchini, ginger, and onion.
2. Cook these for five minutes, and then add in the tomatoes and tofu. Stir around to cook a bit longer.

3. After another 5 minutes, add in the curry powder, salt, water, and coconut milk. Let it simmer for a bit.

4. Ten minutes later, the dish is ready. Stir in the cilantro and enjoy!

Loaded Spaghetti Squash

What's inside:

- Lemon zest (.5 tsp.)
- Torn basil leaves (1 c.)
- Salt (.5 tsp.)
- Oregano (.5 tsp.)
- Brown or green lentils, cooked (1 c.)
- Diced tomatoes (6)
- Minced garlic cloves (1)
- Chopped leek (1)
- Olive oil (1.5 Tbsp.)
- Sliced spaghetti squash (1)

How to make:

1. Turn on the oven and give it some time to heat up to 375 degrees. While that is warming up, add a bit of oil on each half of the spaghetti squash and then place these face down on a baking tray that is lined with parchment paper.

2. Add the squash to the oven and let it bake until it has time to be tender. After half an hour, the dish should be done.

3. While that is cooking, heat up the rest of the oil in a skillet. Add in the tomatoes, garlic, and leak.

4. After eight minutes, you can add in the dried oregano and the lentils, cooking for an additional 5 minutes.

5. When the squash is done, take it out of the oven and use a fork to separate out the flesh.

6. Add the lentil and vegetable mixture to this flesh and combine.

7. Top with the olive oil, lemon zest, and torn basil leaves before serving.

Spicy Pasta

What's inside:

- Torn basil leaves (1 c.)
- Crushed pepper (1 tsp.)
- Salt (1 tsp.)
- Diced chili pepper (1)
- Sliced black olives (.5 c.)
- Diced zucchini (.5)
- Diced sun-dried tomatoes (.5 c.)
- Diced cherry tomatoes (2 c.)

- Diced carrot (1)
- Diced celery stalks (1)
- Diced shallot (1)
- Minced garlic cloves (1)
- Olive oil (3 Tbsp.)
- Spelt pasta (8 oz.)

How to make:

1. Use the instructions on the package to cook up the spelt noodles. Drain out the water and leave to the side.
2. Add some oil to a skillet before cooking the shallot, carrot, celery, and garlic until they are soft.
3. After eight minutes, toss in the zucchini, sun-dried tomatoes, cherry tomatoes, pepper, salt, chili pepper, and olives.
4. When this is done, toss the pasta into the pan and combine well. Move over to a serving plate and top with some basil leaves before serving.

Stuffed Peppers

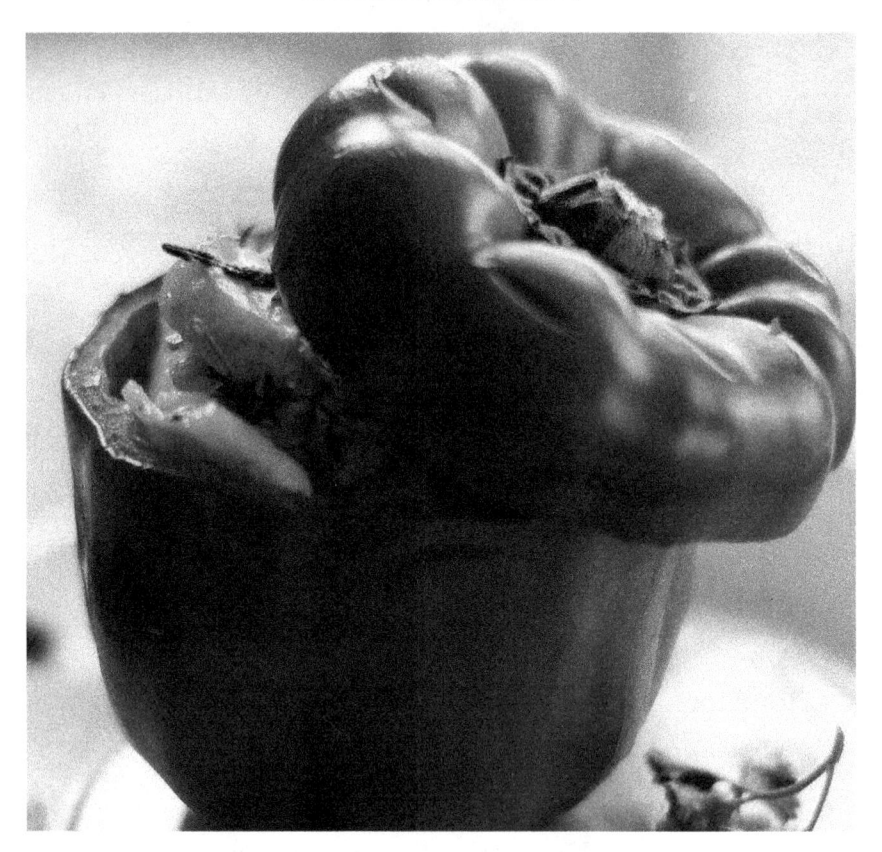

What's inside:

- Bell peppers, tops cut off (2)
- Crushed pepper (1 tsp.)
- Salt (1 tsp.)
- Chopped cilantro (1 Tbsp.)
- Juiced lime (.5)

- Chili powder (1 tsp.)
- Cumin (1 tsp.)
- Olive oil (2 Tbsp.)
- Diced avocado (.5)
- Diced cucumber (1)
- Diced red bell pepper (1)
- Cooked green lentils (.5 c.)
- Cooked quinoa (1 c.)

How to make:

1. Bring out a bowl and combine together the avocado, cucumber, diced bell pepper, lentil, and quinoa.
2. In another bowl, whisk together the salt, cilantro, lime juice, chili, cumin, pepper, and olive oil.
3. Pour this mixture over the lentil and quinoa mixture and stir. Use this mixture to stuff each of the peppers before serving.

Baba Ganoush Pasta

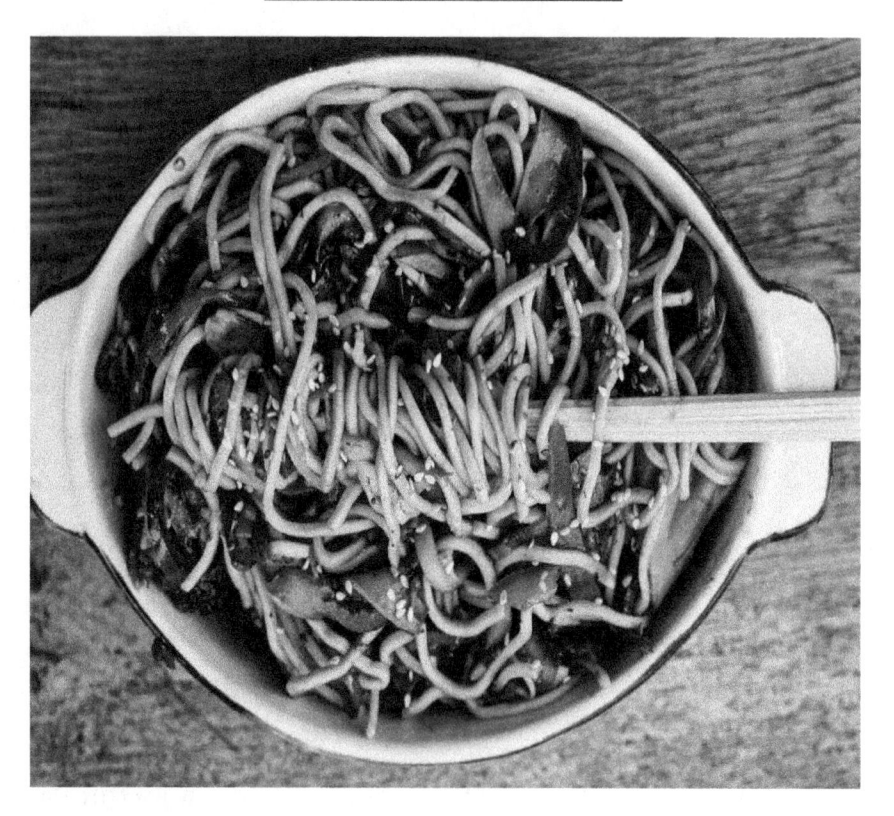

What's inside:

- Chopped parsley (.25 c.)
- Cayenne pepper (1 pinch)
- Salt (.5 tsp.)
- Vegetable stock (1 c.)
- Chopped chili pepper (1)
- Minced garlic clove (1)

- Chopped onion (1)
- Cubed red bell pepper (.5)
- Cubed zucchini (1)
- Cubed eggplant (1)
- Olive oil (1 Tbsp.)
- Spelt pasta (6 oz.)

How to make:

1. Follow the directions on the package to cook up the spelt pasta, and then set it to the side.
2. Heat up some oil in a skillet, and when the oil is ready, add in the chili pepper, garlic, onion, pepper, zucchini, and eggplant to the skillet.
3. After 6 minutes of cooking, add in the vegetable stock and let it cook for another 5 minutes or until warm.
4. Take this from the oven and give it a few minutes to cool down before adding into the blender. Mix until nice and smooth.
5. Add the sauce back to your skillet and season with some of the pepper and salt. Toss in the cooked pasta and sprinkle on the parsley before serving.

Cheesy Broccoli Bowl

What's inside:

- Crushed black pepper (.5 tsp.)
- Salt (.5 tsp.)
- Nutritional yeast (.24 c.)
- Lemon juice (1 Tbsp.)
- Cooked broccoli florets (4 c.)
- Cooked quinoa (1 c.)
- Olive oil (1 tsp.)

How to make:

1. To start this recipe, bring out a skillet and add in the oil, broccoli, and cooked quinoa.
2. After five minutes, this should be nice and warm so add in the pepper, salt, nutritional yeast, and lemon juice.
3. Take the dish off the heat and then serve warm.

Green Bean and Lentil Salad

What's inside:

- Scallion (2 Tbsp.)
- Apple cider vinegar (.25 c.)
- Sliced green beans (2 c.)
- Halved cherry tomatoes (1 c.)
- Cooked green lentils (2 c.)

Pesto Sauce

- Salt (1 tsp.)
- Olive oil (.25 c.)
- Chopped garlic clove (1)
- Pine nuts (2 Tbsp.)
- Spinach (.5 c.)
- Basil leaves (.75 c.)

How to make:

1. Bring out the food processor and add in all of the ingredients for the pesto sauce to make them creamy and smooth.

2. In another bowl, combine together the vinegar, green beans, tomatoes, lentils, and the scallions.

3. Drizzle the pesto sauce over the mixture in the bowl, toss around to coat, and then serve.

Vegetable Minestrone

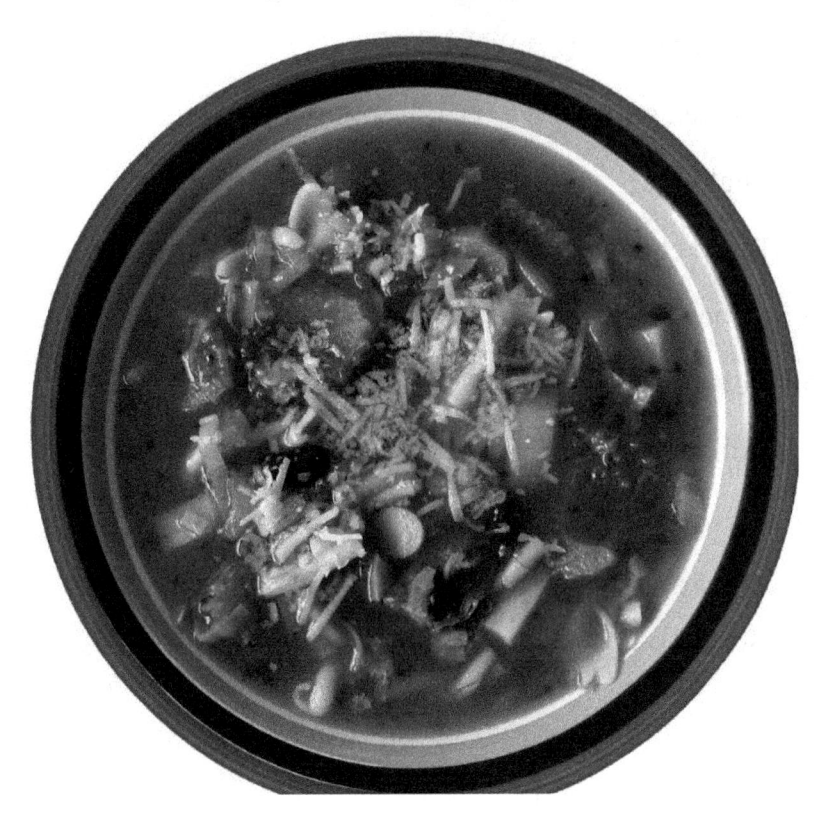

What's inside:

- Spinach (1 c.)
- Basil (1 c.)
- Pepper (1 tsp.)
- Salt (2 tsp.)
- Oregano (1 Tbsp.)
- Diced tomatoes (1 c.)

- Vegetable stock (1 c.)
- Kidney beans (.5 c.)
- Minced garlic clove (1)
- Shallot (1)
- Diced carrot (.5 c.)
- Cubed zucchini (.5 c.)
- Cubed butternut squash (.5 c.)
- Cubed eggplant (.5 c.)
- Olive oil (1 Tbsp.)

How to make:

1. Bring out a bit stock pot and heat up the olive oil inside. When the oil is warm, add the garlic, shallot, carrot, zucchini, squash, and eggplant to the pot.

2. After five minutes for those to cook, add in the salt, oregano, diced tomatoes, stock, kidney beans, and pepper.

3. Let these ingredients simmer together for ten more minutes, adding in more spices if you would like.

4. Stir in the spinach and basil right before serving and enjoy.

Southwest Burger

What's inside:

- Sliced avocado (1)
- Lettuce leaves, Bibb (2)
- Arugula (1 c.)
- Dijon mustard (1 Tbsp.)
- Crushed walnuts (1 Tbsp.)
- Nutritional yeast (1 Tbsp.)
- Firm tofu (4 oz.)
- Crushed black pepper (.5 tsp.)
- Cayenne pepper (.5 tsp.)
- Ground cumin (1 tsp.)
- Salt (1 tsp.)
- Diced carrot (1)
- Diced green bell pepper (1 c.)
- Diced yellow onion (5.)
- Olive oil (1 Tbsp.)

How to make:

1. Heat up some oil in a skillet. When the oil is warm, add in the onion, pepper, cayenne, cumin, salt, carrot, and bell pepper.

2. After five minutes, the vegetables should be soft. Pour them into a bowl and let them cool down.

3. Grate the tofu over the bowl and then add in the Dijon mustard, walnuts, and nutritional yeast. Combine this well and shape into two burgers.

4. Turn on the oven and let it heat up to 400 degrees. Add the burgers on a baking tray that has been lined with paper, and then add to the oven.

5. After half an hour, the burgers should be done. Take them out of the oven and give them time to cool before topping with some avocado and serving.

Zucchini Rolls with Red Sauce

What's inside:

- Basil leaves (15)
- Sliced zucchinis (2)
- Water (.75 c.)
- Dried oregano (1 tsp.)
- Salt (1 tsp.)
- Diced red bell pepper (1)
- Diced Roma tomatoes (3)
- Chopped yellow onion (1)
- Olive oil (1 Tbsp.)

Basil Filling

- Chopped basil (1 handful)
- Nutmeg (.25 tsp.)
- Crushed pepper (.25 tsp.)
- Salt (.5 tsp.)
- Nutritional yeast (1 Tbsp.)
- Water (3 Tbsp.)
- Juiced lemon (1)
- Soaked cashews (1 c.)

How to make:

1. Bring out a skillet and heat up some oil inside. Add in the oregano, salt, bell pepper, tomato, and onion to make your red veggie mixture.

2. Cook for a few minutes to make the vegetables soft, and then add in some water. Let this simmer for a bit.

3. After ten minutes, take the skillet from the heat and give the vegetable mixture some time to cool down.

4. Move over to the blender and then blend until smooth.

5. Now, work on the cashew filling. Clean out the food processor and add in all the ingredients until they are smooth. This can take a bit so be patient to get it done.

6. Place the ribbons of zucchini on a platter in front of you and split up the filling between each one. Roll up each ribbon tightly and then add to a baking dish with the red veggie mixture out on the bottom.

7. Top each of these rolls with the rest of the red veggie mixture and add to the oven that is heated to 375 degrees.

8. After 15 minutes, take the baking dish out of the oven and let the dish cool down. Before serving, top on the basil leaves and enjoy.

Meatless Taco Wraps

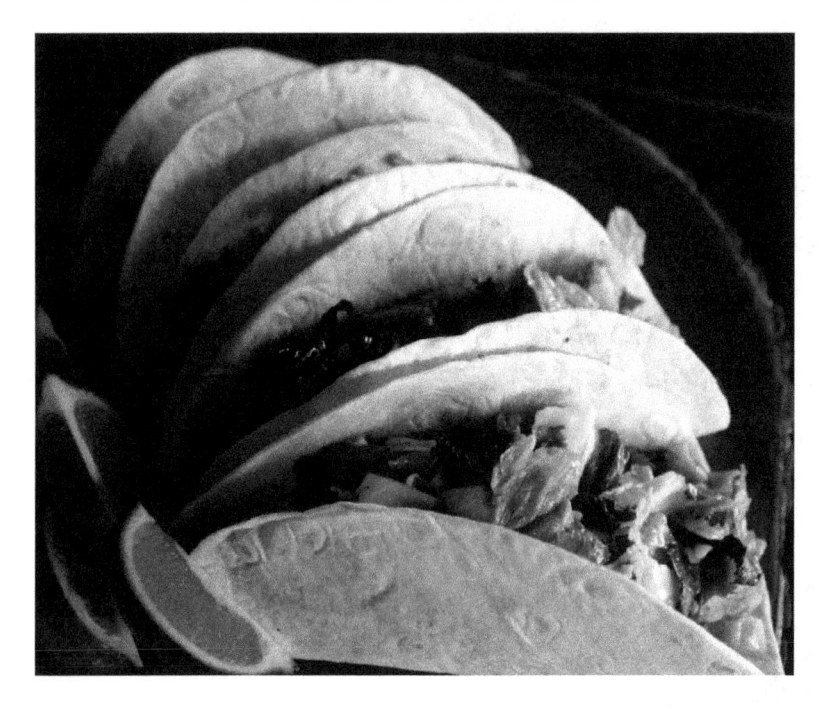

What's inside:

- Sliced avocado (.5)
- Romaine leaves (4)
- Water (.25 c.)
- Salt (.5 tsp.)
- Cumin (.5 tsp.)
- Chili powder (.5 tsp.)
- Smoked paprika (.5 tsp.)
- Minced garlic clove (1)

- Tomato paste (1 Tbsp.)
- Toasted walnuts (.5 c.)
- Cooked brown lentils (1.5 c.)

For the salsa

- Crushed pepper (.5 tsp.)
- Salt (.5 tsp.)
- Apple cider vinegar (1 Tbsp.)
- Chopped cilantro (3 Tbsp.)
- Diced green bell pepper (.5 c.)
- Diced red bell pepper (.5 c.)
- Diced mango (.5 c.)

How to make:

1. Start out with the salsa. Do this by adding all of the ingredients into a bowl and stirring around to combine. Let it marinate for a bit while you work on your taco "meat."

2. Bring out the food processor and pulse together the water, salt, cumin, chili powder, paprika, garlic, tomato paste, walnuts, and lentils. You want this to still be a bit crumbly when you are done.

3. Place the walnut and lentil mixture into each romaine lettuce leaf, and then top with the salsa and the slices of avocado before serving.

Sesame and Quinoa Pilaf

What's inside:

- Cooked green lentils (1 c.)
- Broth or water (1 c.)
- Quinoa (.5 c.)
- Minced garlic clove (1)
- Diced green bell pepper (.5 c.)
- Diced celery stalk (1)
- Sliced shallot (1)
- Crushed pepper (2 tsp.)
- Salt (2 tsp.)
- Olive oil (2 Tbsp.)
- Sliced carrots (2)
- Trimmed and sliced green beans (1 c.)

For the dressing

- Black sesame seeds (2 Tbsp.)
- Rice vinegar (.25 c.)
- Tamari (.25 c.)
- Red chili flakes (.5 tsp.)
- Lemon zest (1 tsp.)

- Grated ginger (1 tsp.)
- Toasted sesame oil (2 tsp.)
- Avocado oil (.33 c.)

How to make:

1. Add the carrots and green beans onto some parchment paper on a baking tray. Drizzle the pepper, salt, and a tablespoon of the olive oil on top.
2. Add to the broiler of the oven and cook until they are browned. This will take about five minutes.
3. After that is done, take out a pot and add in the garlic, bell pepper, celery, shallot, and the rest of the oil inside.
4. Cook the ingredients for five minutes before adding in the quinoa and stirring to cook a bit longer.
5. Now, add in the water or the broth and bring to a boil. Let it simmer for a bit until the liquid is all gone.
6. Now, you can make the dressing. To do this, whisk together all of the ingredients in a bowl to combine.
7. When it is time to assemble, mix together the quinoa and lentils. Season with some pepper and salt and then top with the carrot and bean mixture before drizzling the dressing over the whole thing.

Blackened Salmon with Fruit Salsa

What's inside:

- Mixed greens (4 c.)
- Olive oil (1 Tbsp.)
- Crushed pepper (.25 tsp.)
- Salt (.25 tsp.)
- Chili powder (.5 tsp.)
- Garlic powder (1 tsp.)
- Cayenne pepper (1 tsp.)
- Salmon (8 oz.)

To make the salsa

- Salt
- Chopped cilantro (1 Tbsp.)
- Juiced and zested lime (1)
- Diced pineapple (.5 c.)
- Diced mango (.5 c.)
- Diced green bell pepper (.5)

How to make:

1. Start this recipe by making the mango pineapple salsa. Add all of the ingredients into a bowl and stir to combine. Set aside for now.

2. In another bowl, combine together the pepper, salt, chili powder, garlic powder, and cayenne. Place this mixture out on a flat plate to use in a moment.

3. Heat up a skillet on the stove on medium heat. Brush the olive oil all over the salmon fillet before adding the flesh side to the spice mixture on your plate.

4. Add the flesh side to the pan and let it cook. After five minutes, flip the fish over and cook a bit longer until the fish is all done.

5. Serve the fish with the mixed greens that you chose along with some of the salsa on top.

Arugula Salad with Shrimp

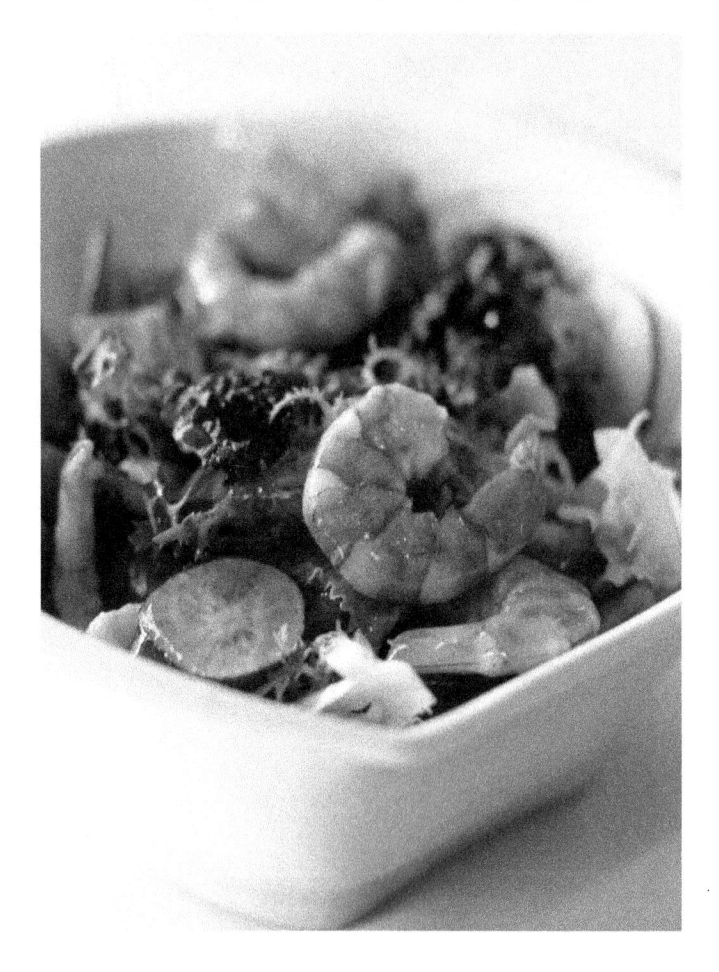

What's inside:

- Crushed black pepper (.5 tsp.)
- Salt (.5 tsp.)
- Chopped parsley (1 Tbsp.)
- Minced garlic clove (1)

- Olive oil (2 Tbsp.)
- Juiced lemon (.5)
- Shrimp (10)

For the salad

- Toasted pine nuts (2 tsp.)
- Salt (1 tsp.)
- Olive oil (2 Tbsp.)
- Juiced lemon (.5)
- Apple cider vinegar (2 Tbsp.)
- Halved cherry tomatoes (10)
- Arugula (4 c.)

How to make:

1. Take out a bowl and add in the pepper, parsley, salt, garlic, olive oil, lemon juice, and shrimp inside. Place into the fridge to marinate for fifteen minutes or more.
2. When you are ready, take out a skillet and heat it up. Add the prepared shrimp inside and cook for a bit on each side until the shrimp is all cooked through.
3. Now, it is time to make the salad. Bring out a big salad bowl and combine together all of the ingredients for the salad together.
4. Add the shrimp on top of the salad and then serve warm.

Easy Pizza

What's inside:

- Lemon juice (1 tsp.)
- Salt (1 tsp.)
- Nutritional yeast (2 Tbsp.)
- Olive oil (2 tsp.)
- Arugula (1 c.)
- Sliced tomato (1)
- Sliced avocado (1)

For the dough

- Dried basil (1 tsp.)
- Dried oregano (1 tsp.)
- Pepper (1 tsp.)
- Salt (1 tsp.)
- Olive oil (4 Tbsp.)
- Minced garlic clove (1)
- Ground flaxseeds (.33 c.)
- Sunflower seeds, soaked (1.25 c.)

How to make:

1. Bring out a blender and pulse the sunflower seeds a few times. Then add them into a big bowl along with the basil, oregano, salt, pepper, olive oil, garlic, and flaxseed flour.

2. Knead this mixture together until you get a nice dough to form. You can add in some more water if needed.

3. Roll the dough out into the shape of a pizza. Add some parchment paper to your baking tray and put the dough on top.

4. Heat your oven to the lowest temperature that it allows and then place the baking tray inside to dehydrate the dough. Give this about 12 hours to finish up.

5. When the dough is ready, you can layer on the tomato slices and avocado on the crust.

6. Toss the arugula into a small bowl with the lemon juice, salt, nutritional yeast, and olive oil. Place this on top of the pizza and serve the whole thing right away.

Chapter 9

Snack Recipes for Easy Snacking

Watercress and Endive Boats

What's inside:
- Watercress (1 c.)
- Endive leaves (10)
- Salt (1 tsp.)
- Garlic clove (1)
- Lemon juice (1 Tbsp.)
- Mint (.25 c.)
- Parsley (.5 c.)
- Avocado (1)
- Spinach (3 c.)

How to make:
1. Take all of your ingredients except for the watercress and endive leaves and add them into a blender.
2. Add the lid on top of the blender and mix those ingredients together until they are smooth and form a nice dip.

3. Scoop this dip that you just made into each of the endive leaves before topping with the watercress and enjoying!

Toasted Trail mix

What's inside:

- Salt
- Toasted pepitas (1 Tbsp.)
- Raisins (2 Tbsp.)
- Toasted almonds (2 Tbsp.)
- Toasted walnuts (3 Tbsp.)
- Toasted coconut chips (3 Tbsp.)

How to make:

1. Add all of the ingredients into a bag or another storage container and shake around to combine.
2. Divide into two or three portions and enjoy.

Avocado Chickpea Cups

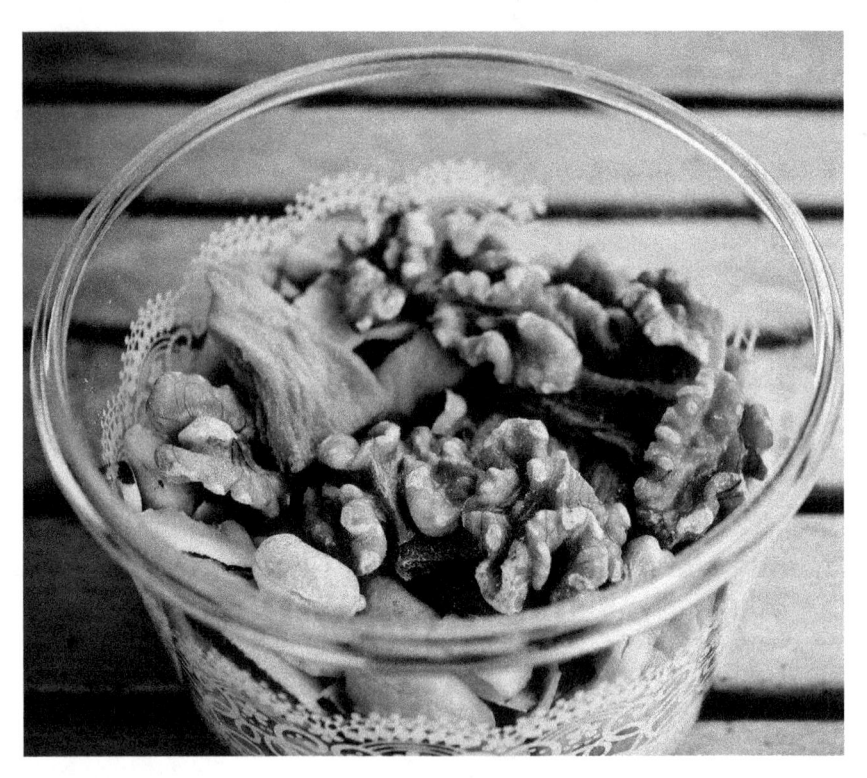

What's inside:

- Oregano (1 tsp.)
- Chopped basil (1 Tbsp.)
- Crushed black pepper (.5 tsp.)
- Salt (.5 tsp.)
- Lemon juice (1 Tbsp.)
- Olive oil (2 Tbsp.)

- Diced shallot (1)
- Diced tomato (.5)
- Cooked chickpeas (.5 c.)
- Ripe avocado (1)

How to make:

1. To start this recipe, bring out a bowl and combine the pepper, salt, lemon juice, olive oil, shallot, tomato, and chickpeas.
2. Set this mixture aside and let it rest for about five minutes.
3. In the meantime, slice up the avocado going in half lengthwise before taking the pit out of it.
4. Spoon the tomato and chickpea mixture in the middle of the avocados. Garnish with the basil and oregano before serving.

Cocoa Truffles with Spice

What's inside:

- Cayenne pepper (.25 tsp.)
- Salt (.25 tsp.)
- Raw cacao powder (6 Tbsp.)
- Unsweetened coconut (.33 c.)
- Almond meal (.5 c.)
- Pitted dates (2 c.)

How to make:

1. Bring out your food processor and pulse to combine the shredded coconut, almond meal, and dates until they are crumbly.
2. Add in half the cacao along with the cayenne and sea salt. Blend this together until you get a sticky paste that is able to form into a ball.
3. Tear off pieces of the dough and shape into six even-sized balls.
4. Place the rest of your cacao on a plate and roll each of the balls lightly through this. Store or eat right away.

Zesty Chips

What's inside:

- Nutritional yeast (2 Tbsp.)

- Chili powder (1 tsp.)
- Cayenne pepper (1 tsp.)
- Crushed black pepper (1 tsp.)
- Salt (1 tsp.)
- Olive oil (1 Tbsp.)
- Sliced kale (1 bunch)

How to make:

1. Turn on the oven and let it have time to reach 300 degrees. Use some parchment paper to line two baking trays.

2. While the oven is heating up, add the kale to a large bowl and pour the olive oil on tap. Use your hands to massage the oil on the kale until it is coated.

3. In another bowl, combine together the nutritional yeast, chili powder, cayenne, pepper, and salt.

4. Sprinkle this over the kale, making sure that the spices get all over the kale. Then, pour this in an even layer on the baking tray and put into the oven.

5. After 10 minutes, flip the chips over and allow them to cook for a bit longer.

6. After another 10 minutes, take the chips out of the oven and give them some time to cool down before serving.

Summer Fruit Soup

What's inside:

- Raspberries (4)
- Chopped mint leaves (1 Tbsp.)
- Salt (.25 tsp.)
- Raw honey (1 Tbsp.)
- Water (.5 c.)
- Coconut milk (1 c.)
- Lime juice (2 Tbsp.)
- Cubed honeydew (1 c.)
- Cubed watermelon (1 c.)
- Cubed cantaloupe (1 c.)

How to make:

1. To start this recipe, bring out the food processor and add in the salt, honey, water, coconut milk, lime juice, honeydew, watermelon, and cantaloupe.
2. Pulse these together until you get it nice and combined into a fruit liquid.
3. Pour this into a bowl and add to the fridge to chill. After 60 minutes, you can garnish this dish with the raspberries and mint before serving.

Maple Roasted Carrots

What's inside:

- Toasted sesame seeds (1 Tbsp.)
- Crushed pepper (.25 tsp.)
- Salt (1 tsp.)
- Lemon zest (1 tsp.)
- Maple syrup (1 Tbsp.)
- Melted ghee (1 Tbsp.)
- Carrot sliced (3)

How to make:

1. Turn on the oven and let it heat up to 400 degrees. Then take out a small bowl and whisk together the pepper, salt, lemon zest, maple syrup, and ghee.

2. Add the carrots into a baking dish and coat with the maple and ghee mixture that you just made. Add to the oven.

3. After 25 minutes, and turning the carrots halfway through, you can take them out of the oven and give them a few minutes to cool down.

4. Before serving, sprinkle on the sesame seeds before enjoying.

Smokey Caesar Salad

What's inside:

- Salt (.5 tsp.)
- Honey (1 tsp.)
- Filtered water (1.25 c.)
- Nutritional yeast (1 Tbsp.)
- Garlic cloves (2)
- Smoked paprika (.5 tsp.)
- Chipotle powder (.25 tsp.)
- Almonds (.33 c.)
- Diced cucumber (.5)
- Halved cherry tomatoes (5)
- Pumpkin seeds (1 c.)
- Kale, sliced (1 bunch)

How to make:

1. Bring out your blender and combine together the salt, honey, water, nutritional yeast, garlic, smoked paprika, chipotle powder, and the almonds.

2. Place the cucumber, cherry tomatoes, pumpkin seeds, and kale into a big bowl.

3. Pour the dressing that you made in the blender over the vegetables, tossing well to allow all of the leaves of the salad to become coated.

4. Let the salad set for a minute or two before serving.

Spicy Mix with Tortilla Chips

What's inside:

- Corn tortilla chips (24)
- Olive oil (1 Tbsp.)
- Juiced lime (1)
- Red chili flakes (.25 tsp.)
- Cayenne pepper (.5 tsp.)
- Salt (.5 tsp.)
- Chopped cilantro (2 Tbsp.)
- Diced jalapeno (1)
- Grated garlic cloves (2)
- Sliced green onions (2)
- Diced green bell pepper (1)
- Diced tomatoes (3)

How to make:

1. Take out a bowl and combine together all of the ingredients except for your tortilla chips.

2. Add half of this mixture into the blender or a food processor, and then pulse it 10 times.
3. Pour this mixture back into the original bowl with the rest of the ingredients, making sure to stir to combine.
4. Add to the fridge to chill for half an hour or longer before serving with the tortilla chips.

Creamy Broccoli Soup

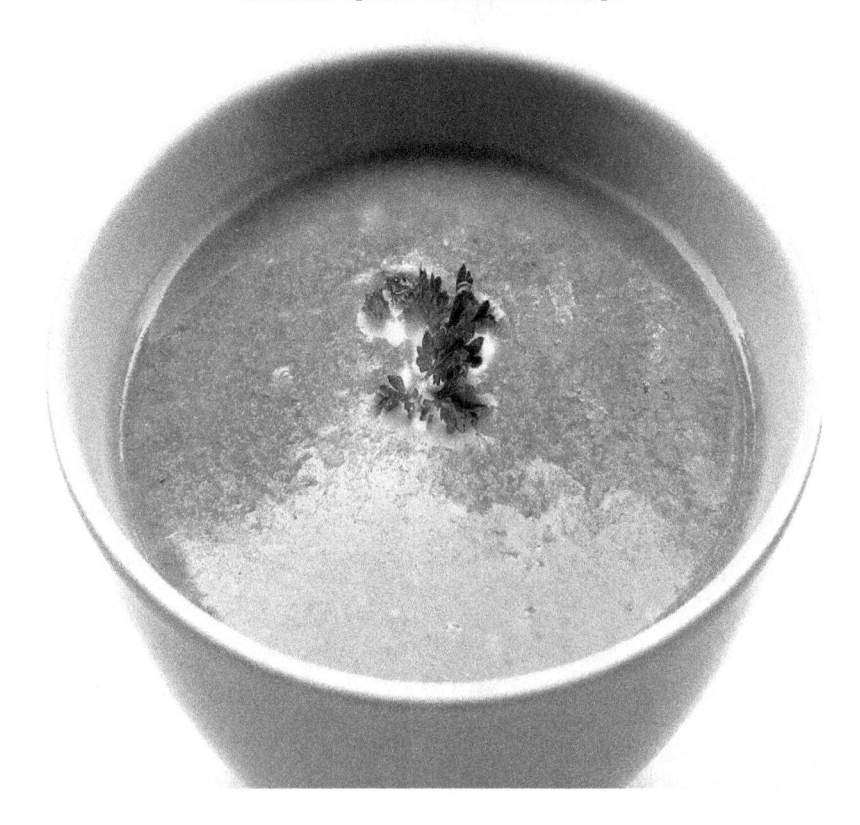

What's inside:

- Crushed black pepper (.5 tsp.)

- Nutmeg (.5 tsp.)
- Salt (1 tsp.)
- Coconut milk (.5 c.)
- Vegetable broth (1 c.)
- Coconut oil (1 Tbsp.)
- Diced shallot (1)
- Avocado (1)
- Broccoli head (1)

How to make:

1. Take out a pan and heat up your oil on the stove. When the oil has time to warm up, add in the broccoli and shallot and cook for a bit.

2. After 10 minutes, pour in your coconut milk and vegetable broth, bringing this all to a simmer.

3. After fifteen minutes, give the mixture time to cool, and then add it to a blender or a food processor, along with your avocado. Blend these ingredients until they are smooth.

4. Add the mixture back to the pan and let it reach a simmer again. Stir in the pepper, salt, and nutmeg before serving warm.

Tortilla Soup

What's inside:

- Diced avocado (1)
- Toasted tortilla wrap, sprouted (1)
- Crushed black pepper (.25 tsp.)
- Salt (.25 tsp.)
- Juiced and zested lime (1)
- Chopped spinach (1 c.)
- Chopped cilantro (1 c.)
- Vegetable broth (1 c.)
- Water (1 c.)
- Red chili flakes (1 tsp.)
- Cayenne pepper (1 tsp.)
- Cumin (1 tsp.)
- Diced tomato (1)
- Diced red bell pepper (1)
- Diced jalapeno (1)
- Diced shallot (1)
- Olive oil (1 Tbsp.)

How to make:

1. Take out a big pot and heat up some olive oil on medium-low heat. When the oil is warm, add in the tomato, red bell pepper, jalapeno, and shallot to cook.
2. After five minutes, add in the chili flakes, cayenne pepper, and cumin and stir to warm up before adding in the vegetable broth and water.
3. Let all of the ingredients come to a boil. When the boil is reached, reduce the heat and let it simmer for 15 minutes.
4. Reduce the heat before adding in the pepper, salt, lime juice, lime zest, cilantro, and spinach.
5. Place in some bowls to serve with the avocado and tortilla strips on top!

Alkaline Gazpacho

What's inside:
- Green onions (2 Tbsp.)
- Crushed pepper (.25 tsp.)
- Salt (.25 tsp.)
- Cayenne pepper (.5 tsp.)
- Cumin (.5 tsp.)
- Paprika (.5 tsp.)
- Chopped cilantro (1 Tbsp.)
- Diced shallot (1)
- Diced cucumber (.5)

- Water (1 c.)
- Vegetable broth (1 c.)
- Pitted avocado (1)
- Juiced lemon (1)
- Seeded and chopped jalapeno (.5)
- Chopped cilantro (.5 c.)
- Chopped parsley (1 c.)
- Olive oil (1 Tbsp.)
- Chopped green bell pepper (1)
- Tomatoes (1)

How to make:

1. To start this recipe, bring out your blender and get it all set up. Add in all of the ingredients besides the green onions into the blender.
2. Place the lid on top and then mix the ingredients together until they are smooth and combined.
3. Move this to the fridge to chill for about two hours. When you are ready to serve, pour into some bowls and garnish with the green peppers.

Butternut Squash Soup

What's inside:

- Almond milk (.25 c.)
- Nutmeg (.25 tsp.)
- Crushed pepper (1 tsp.)
- Salt (1 tsp.)
- Maple syrup (1 Tbsp.)
- Vegetable broth (3 c.)
- Sage leaves (5)
- Peeled and cubed butternut squash (1)
- Minced garlic clove (1)
- Sliced shallots (2)
- Olive oil (3 Tbsp.)

How to make:

1. Bring out a saucepan and heat it up on the stove. Add in two tablespoons of the oil along with the garlic and shallot to cook.
2. After five minutes, add in the nutmeg, pepper, salt, maple syrup broth, three sage leaves, and the butternut squash.
3. Bring this mixture up so that it boils before reducing the heat and simmering for 20 minutes or until you notice that the squash is soft.

4. Turn the heat off and give the mixture some time to cool down. When it is cool enough, add the mixture to a blender and combine to make smooth.

5. Pour the mixture back into a pan and then bring to a simmer. Add in the almond milk and continue to cook for another three minutes.

6. Taking out another small pan, add in the rest of the oil. When it is warm, add in the rest of the sage leaves.

7. After four minutes, take the sage leaves out and set them to the side. Pour this into serving bowls and top with the frizzled sage leaves before enjoying.

Chilled Tomato Soup

What's inside:

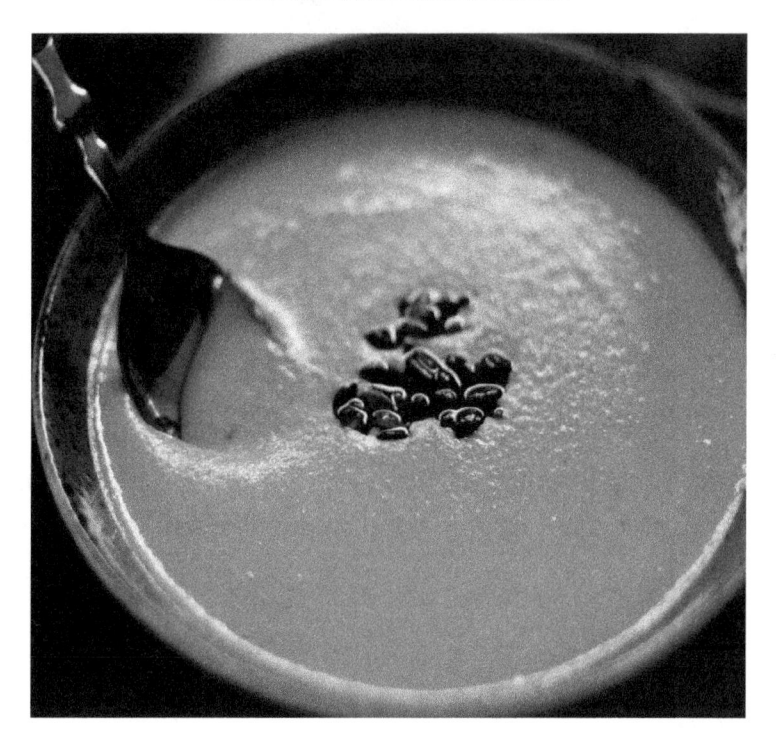

- Sugar-free hot sauce (1 tsp.)
- Chopped parsley (1.5 Tbsp.)
- Olive oil (1 Tbsp.)
- Tamari (1 tsp.)
- Cumin (1 tsp.)
- Diced jalapeno (1)
- Sliced shallots (2)

- Diced cucumber (1.5)
- Lemon juice (1.5 Tbsp.)
- Apple cider vinegar (1.5 Tbsp.)
- Chopped green bell pepper (.5)
- Peeled tomatoes (3)

How to make:

1. To start this recipe, take out a blender and add all of the ingredients inside to mix well.
2. Add in more water to this if you would like a soup that is a bit thinner, but choose what works the best for you.
3. Add to the fridge for a few hours before serving.

Baked Sweet Potato Fries with BBQ Sauce

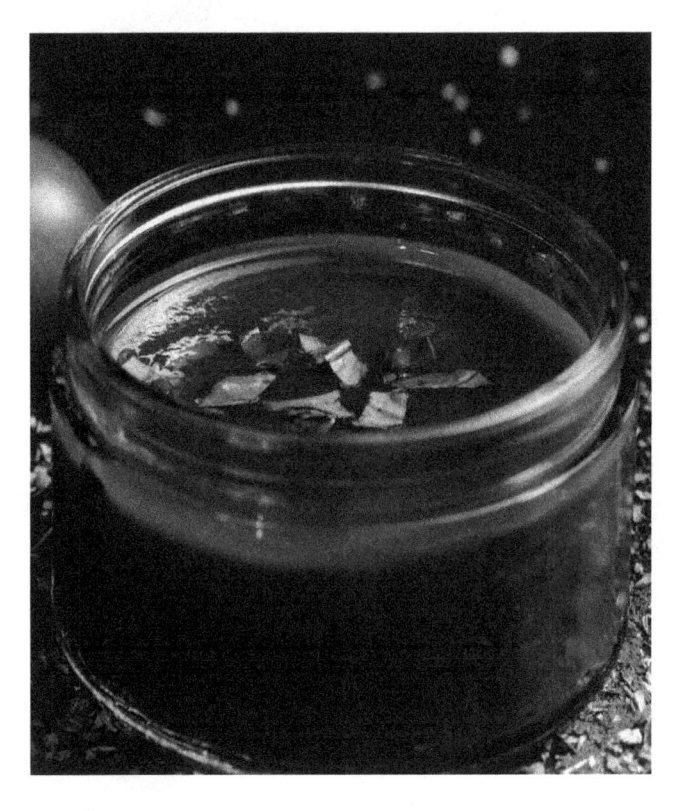

What's inside:

- Garlic powder (.5 tsp.)
- Salt (.5 tsp.)
- Avocado oil (1 Tbsp.)
- Sweet potatoes (1)

For the BBQ sauce

- Cayenne pepper (.5 tsp.)

- Chili powder (1tsp.)
- Smoked paprika (1 tsp.)
- Tamari (1 tsp.)
- Coconut aminos (1 Tbsp.)
- Maple syrup (1 Tbsp.)
- Water (1 Tbsp.)
- Tomato paste (2 Tbsp.)

How to make:

1. First, we need to work on making the BBQ sauce. To do this, bring out a blender and add all of the ingredients for the sauce inside. Blend until nice and smooth.
2. Turn on the oven and give it time to heat up to 400 degrees. While the oven is heating up, toss your sweet potato with the garlic powder, salts, and oil.
3. Place in a single layer on a baking tray lined with parchment paper and put into the oven.
4. After twenty minutes, and flipping the fries halfway through, the potatoes will be done. Server with the BBQ sauce and enjoy.

Eggplant and Cashew Bites

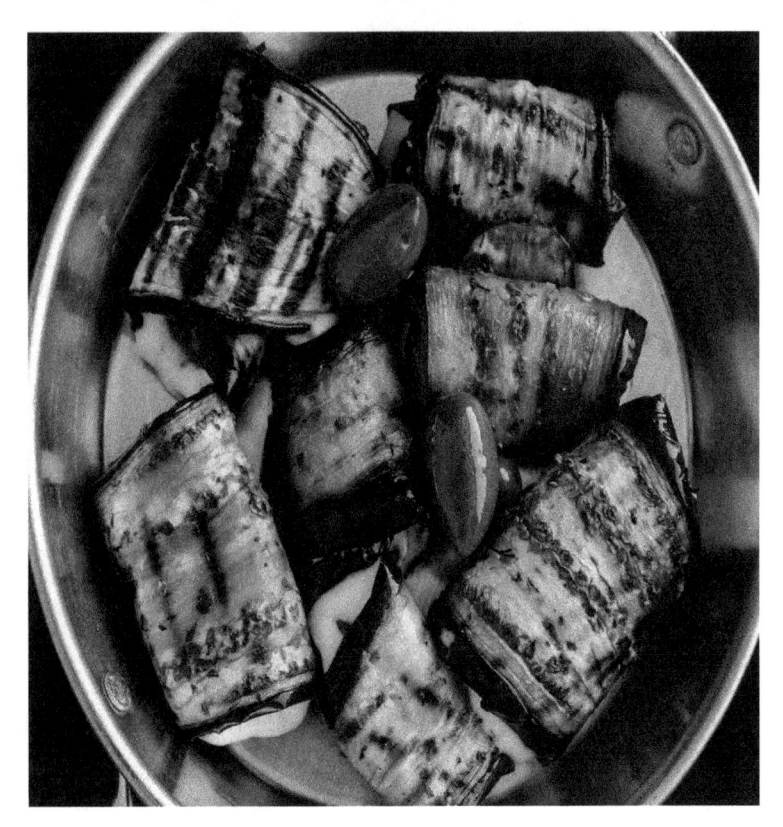

What's inside:

- Raisins (1 Tbsp.)
- Pine nuts (1 Tbsp.)
- Salt (1 tsp.)
- Olive oil (1Tbsp.)
- Sliced eggplant (1)

For the cashew basil filling

- Chopped basil (1 handful)
- Nutmeg (.25 tsp.)
- Crushed pepper (.25 tsp.)
- Salt (.5 tsp.)
- Nutritional yeast (1 Tbsp.)
- Water (3 Tbsp.)
- Juiced lemon (1)
- Soaked cashews (1 c.)

How to make:

1. Turn on the broiler and give it time to heat up. While the broiler is warming up, line a baking tray with some parchment paper to set up.
2. Brush each piece of the eggplant with some of the oil and season with salt. Add to the baking tray and then into the oven.
3. After four minutes, flip the eggplant over and then bake a bit longer.
4. Now, you can work on the cashew basil filling. Place all of the ingredients into the food processor until they become smooth.
5. Take this filling out of the food processor and mix in the raisins and the pine nuts.

6. Add a bit of this filling on top of each slip of eggplant and roll it up. Secure with a toothpick and then serve.

Chapter 10

Dessert Recipes to End the Day

Cookie Dough Bites

What's inside:
- Cacao nibs (2 Tbsp.)
- Cooked chickpeas (.5 c.)
- Cacao powder, raw (.25 c.)
- Melted coconut oil (2 Tbsp.)
- Maple syrup (3 Tbsp.)
- Vanilla (1 Tbsp.)
- Cinnamon (.25 tsp.)
- Salt (.5 tsp.)
- Raw almonds (1 c.)
- Oats (1 c.)

How to make:
1. Take out the food processor and add in the vanilla, cinnamon, salt, almonds, and oats.

2. Blend these until they make flour, and then add in the chickpeas, cacao, coconut oil, and maple syrup. Continue to blend until a nice dough starts to form.

3. Stir in the cacao nibs and then form these into smaller balls. Add into the fridge to chill for a few hours before serving.

Cashew Chip Cookies

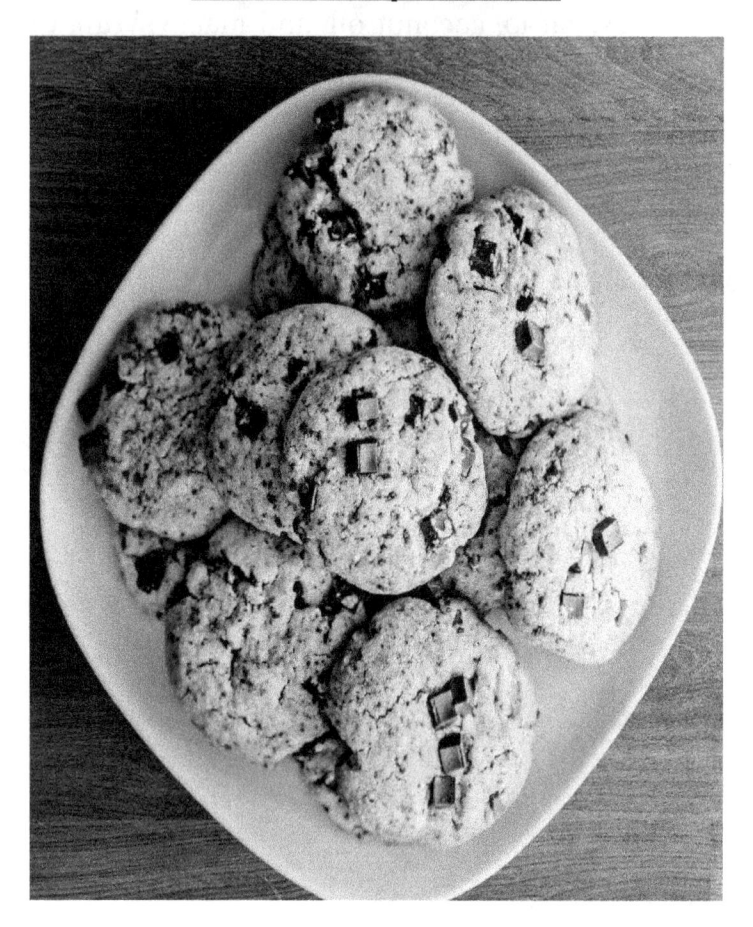

What's inside:

- Chocolate chips, vegan (.33 c.)
- Salt (.25 tsp.)
- Baking powder (.5 tsp.)
- Honey (.25 c.)

- Cashew butter (.25 c.)
- Vanilla (1 tsp.)
- Garbanzo beans (.5 can)

How to make:

1. Turn on the oven and allow it time to heat up to 350 degrees. While the oven is heating up, take out a baking tray and line it with some parchment paper.
2. Put all of the ingredients except for the chocolate chips into your food processor and then blend until it is smooth.
3. Roll the dough into 5 balls and then press down with a fork on the baking tray. Add into the oven to heat up.
4. After 15 minutes, the cookies should be done. Take them out and give them some time to cool down before serving.

Lemon Cookies

What's inside:

- Lemon zest (1 tsp.)
- Coconut butter (1 Tbsp.)
- Lemon juice (1.5 Tbsp.)
- Shredded coconut (1 c. and 2 Tbsp.)
- Pitted and soaked dates (4)
- Almond meal (.5 c.)
- Cashews (.33 c.)

How to make:

1. Start this recipe by taking out the food processor and placing the cashews inside. Pulse these until you are able to get a flour-like texture to form.
2. When this happens, add in the coconut butter, lemon juice, cup of coconut, and almond meal. Continue to process until you get nice dough to form.
3. On a small plate, combine together the lemon zest with the rest of the coconut.
4. Roll the dough into small balls and then roll each of these into the lemon and coconut mixture.
5. Place these into a container or on a plate and add to the fridge to chill for 60 minutes or more.

Lemon Lime Jelly

What's inside:

- Diced kiwi (.5 c.)
- Lemon zest (.5 tsp.)
- Lemon zest (.5 tsp.)
- Honey (1 Tbsp.)
- Lemon extract (.25 tsp.)
- Lime extract (.25 tsp.)
- Coconut milk (.25 c.)
- Water (.25 c.)
- Agar agar powder (.25 tsp.)

How to make:

1. Take out a pan and allow half the water to dissolve the agar agar. Let it stand for about five minutes.
2. While this mixture is standing, heat up the coconut milk in a pan with the heat on low. Five minutes later, heat up the agar agar mixture, making sure to stir the whole time.
3. When this mixture has time to boil, pour the warmed lemon and lime zest, honey, lemon and lime extract, and coconut milk inside.
4. Stir this all together well and let it cook for a few minutes. After this time, take the dessert from the heat and pour into the mold or dish of your choice.

5. Allow this to chill in the fridge for 60 minutes or more. Take out of the mold at this time and top with some of the kiwis before serving.

Strawberry Lime Bites

What's inside:
- Strawberries (6)
- Melted coconut butter (.25 c.)
- Salt (.25 tsp.)
- Lime zest (2 tsp.)
- Shredded coconut (6 Tbsp.)

How to make:
1. Bring out a small plate and combine together the salt, lime zest, and shredded coconut.
2. Take a small amount of the coconut butter and press it against one strawberry, spreading it all around using your fingers.
3. Then roll the fruit all through your lime and coconut mixture. Repeat with the rest of the strawberries.
4. Set the strawberries on a plate and into the fridge for half an hour or more. Then serve when ready.

Coconut Chip Bites

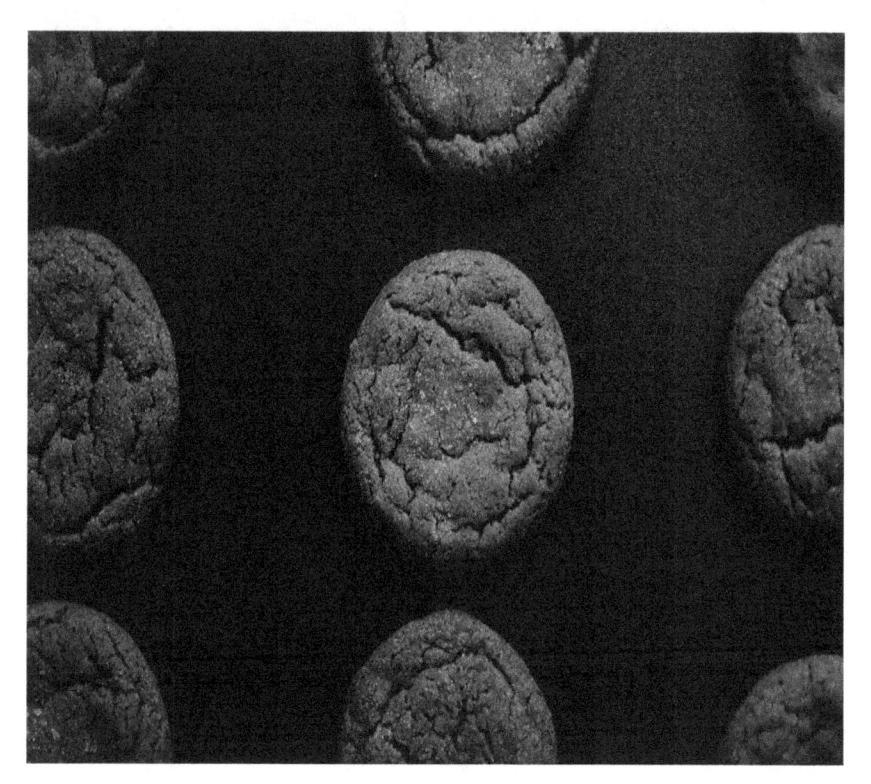

What's inside:

- Cacao nibs (1 tsp.)
- Salt (.25 tsp.)
- Vanilla (.25 tsp.)
- Coconut flour (1 tsp.)
- Shredded coconut (.66 c.)
- Mashed banana (1)

How to make:

1. Turn on the oven and let it heat up to 350 degrees. While the oven is heating up, add some parchment paper to a baking tray.

2. Combine all of your ingredients into a big bowl. Mix this all the way until you get nice dough going.

3. Spoon this into 6 balls and then add them to your prepared tray. Press down on each ball.

4. Add to the oven and let them bake. After 10 minutes, the cookies should be done. Take them out of the oven and allow them some time to cool down first.

Sweet Potato Orange Cookies

What's inside:

- Raisins (1 Tbsp.)
- Orange zest (1 tsp.)
- Salt (.25 tsp.)
- Baking soda (.25 tsp.)
- Baking powder (.25 tsp.)
- Nutmeg (.25 tsp.)
- Cinnamon (.25 tsp.)
- Vanilla (.25 tsp.)
- Orange blossom water (1 tsp.)
- Honey (1.5 Tbsp.)
- Egg (1)
- Cashew butter (1 Tbsp.)
- Quick oats (.33 c.)
- Mashed sweet potato (.75 c.)

How to make:

1. Turn on the oven and let it heat up to 350 degrees. While the oven is heating up, take out a baking tray and line it with some parchment paper.

2. Take out a food processor and add in all of your ingredients besides the raisins inside.

3. Blend the ingredients until they are well combined and then fold the raisins into the mixture as well.

4. Scoop up 12 balls of dough onto the baking tray and flatten with a fork. Add to the oven to bake.

5. After 10 minutes, flip the cookies around. Allow to cook a bit longer, another ten minutes, and then take out of the oven.

6. After a few minutes to cool down, serve the cookies warm.

Cashew Cold Cookies

What's inside:

- Salt (.25 tsp.)
- Cacao nibs (1 tsp.)
- Maple syrup (2 Tbsp.)
- Cashew butter (.33 c.)
- Ground cashews (2 Tbsp.)
- Ground flaxseed (1 Tbsp.)
- Gluten-free rolled oats (.33 c.)
- Shredded coconut (.33 c.)

How to make:

1. Take out a big bowl and combine all of the ingredients above until you get a nice dough forms.
2. Take that dough and use it to make 10 balls. Put these on a plate and then into the fridge.
3. After half an hour or more of the balls chilling, take them out and serve!

Pumpkin Cups

What's inside:
- Crushed pecans (1 Tbsp.)
- Shredded coconut (1 tsp.)
- Ground flaxseed (1 tsp.)
- Vanilla (.5 tsp.)
- Pumpkin puree (.5 c.)
- Maple syrup (1 Tbsp.)
- Ground nutmeg (.25 tsp.)
- Ground cinnamon (.5 tsp.)
- Ground ginger (.5 tsp.)
- Chia seeds (2 Tbsp.)
- Almond milk (1 c.)

How to make:

1. Take all of the ingredients, besides the pecans and the coconut, and add them into a jar with a cover. Shake or stir to combine these ingredients together well.

2. Place a lid or another covering on the jar and place into the fridge. After eight hours, you can take these out.

3. Garnish the pumpkin cups with some pecans and coconut before serving and enjoying.

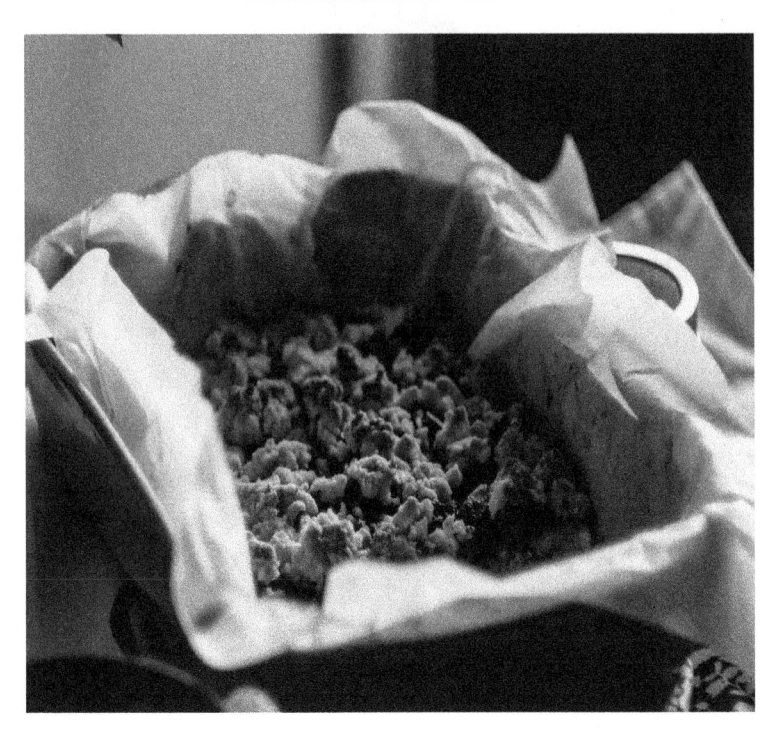

Apricot Crumble

What's inside:

- Cinnamon (.25 tsp.)
- Salt (.5 tsp.)

- Coconut oil (.25 c.)
- Maple syrup (.25 c.)
- Shredded coconut (.25 c.)
- Sunflower seeds (1 Tbsp.)
- Sliced almonds (.25 c.)
- Ground almonds (.5 c.)
- Rolled oats (1 c.)
- Honey (1 Tbsp.)
- Grated ginger (1 Tbsp.)
- Chia seeds (1 Tbsp.)
- Raspberries (.5 c.)
- Chopped apricots (5)
- Coconut oil (1 Tbsp.)

How to make:

1. Turn on the oven and let it heat up to 350 degrees. Take a small baking dish made of glass out and grease it up with a bit of the coconut oil before starting.
2. Bring out a bowl and combine together the apricots and raspberries along with the honey, ginger, and chia seeds.
3. Pour this into your baking dish and then set it to the side.

4. Bring out another bowl and add in the cinnamon, salt, .25 cup of coconut oil, maple syrup, coconut, sunflower seeds, sliced almonds, ground almonds, and oats together.

5. Combine so that the whole mixture is moistened with the syrup and the oil. Sprinkle this over the fruit mixture and add to the oven.

6. After half an hour, take the dish out and give it some time to cool down before serving.

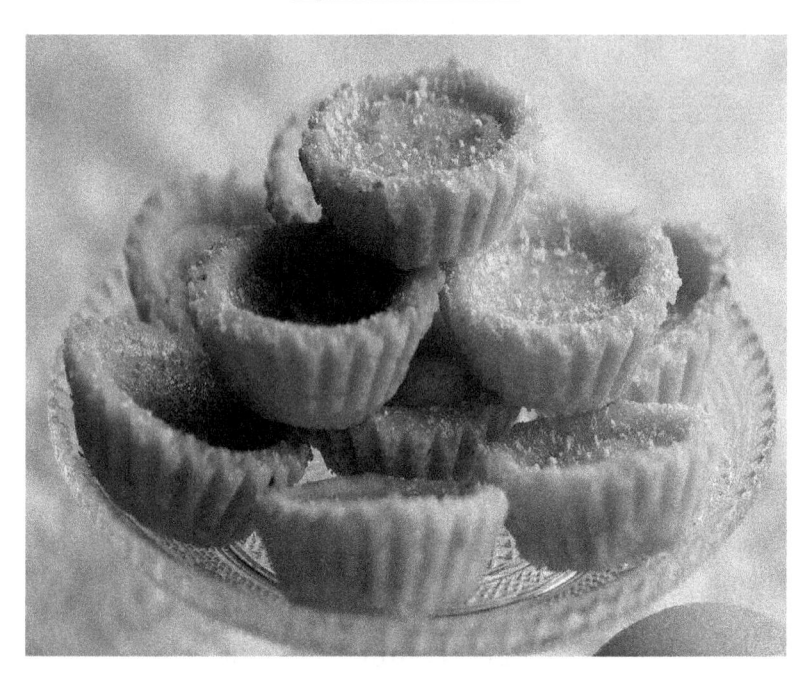

Apricot Tarts

What's inside:

- Mint leaves (8)
- Sliced apricots (2)

- Salt (.5 tsp.)
- Cinnamon (1 tsp.)
- Nutmeg (1 tsp.)
- Dried dates, soaked (.75 c.)
- Raw almonds (.5 c.)

For the cashew filling

- Salt (.5 tsp.)
- Raw honey (1 tsp.)
- Vanilla (1 tsp.)
- Water (3 Tbsp.)
- Lemon zest (.5 Tbsp.)
- Lemon juice (3 Tbsp.)
- Soaked cashews (.5 c.)

How to make:

1. First, we need to look at how to make the shell dough for the tarts. Do this by combining the salt, cinnamon, nutmeg, dried dates, and almonds in a food processor.
2. Pulse this mixture until it turns crumbly and continue to blend until you get a ball to form.
3. Take the dough out of the food processor and form into 8 equal-sized balls. Pressure down in each one into a tart pan, making it even on all sides.

4. Add this to the fridge to chill for ten minutes or more. Then take the shells out of the pan.

5. Using a clean food processor, combine all of the ingredients for the cashew filling until they are smooth. Place in a bowl and then chill for at least ten minutes.

6. In each shell, add the cashew filling and then top with a mint leave and two apricot slices before serving.

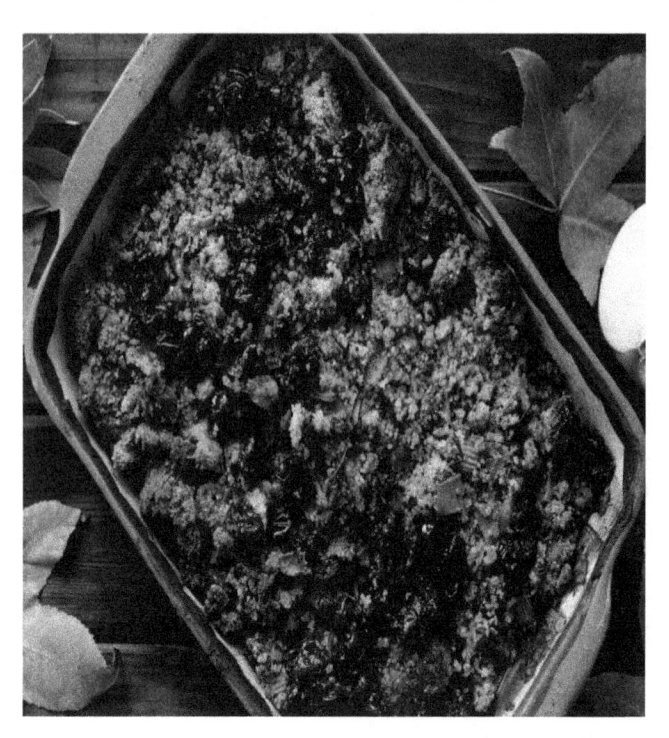

Raw Berry Crumble

What's inside:

- Vanilla (.25 tsp.)
- Salt (.25 tsp.)

- Lime juice (2 tsp.)
- Soaked dates (2)
- Mixed berries (.5 c.)
- Raspberries (.33 c.)
- Blackberries (.33 c.)
- Blueberries (.33 c.)

For the crumble

- Salt (.25 tsp.)
- Nutmeg (.25 tsp.)
- Cinnamon (1 tsp.)
- Dried coconut (.25 c.)
- Dates, soaked (.5 c.)
- Walnuts (.5 c.)
- Pecans (.5 c.)

Whipped coconut cream

- Maple syrup (1 Tbsp.)
- Lemon zest (.5 tsp.)
- Vanilla (.5 tsp.)
- Coconut milk (1 can)

How to make:

1. Bring out the food processor and place the raspberries, blackberries, and blueberries into the food processor along with the vanilla, salt, lime juice, and dates.

2. Blend these ingredients together until combined well. Toss together this fruit mixture with the rest of the mixed berries in a small bowl. Spread this out into the bottom of a glass dish.

3. Clean out the food processor and add in all of the ingredients to the crumble part. Pulse to combine and stop when it reaches the right crumbly texture.

4. Add this mixture over the fruit mixture as well.

5. To make the whipped coconut cream, open up the coconut milk and drain out the water. Add into a bowl and then mix with the maple syrup, lemon zest, and vanilla.

6. Beat the ingredients with a hand mixer for a few minutes until nice and fluffy and then spoon over the crumble.

7. Set in the fridge to chill for about an hour or so and then serve.

Raspberry Cheesecakes

What's inside:

- Raspberries (8)
- Salt (.5 tsp.)
- Cinnamon (1 tsp.)
- Nutmeg (1 tsp.)

- Soaked dates (.75 c.)
- Raw almonds (.5 c.)

Cheesecake filling

- Salt (.5 tsp.)
- Raw honey (1 tsp.)
- Almond extract (.25 tsp.)
- Vanilla (1 tsp.)
- Raspberries (.5 c.)
- Water (3 Tbsp.)
- Lemon zest (.5 Tbsp.)
- Lemon juice (3 Tbsp.)
- Soaked raw cashews (.5 c.)

How to make:

1. Work by making the dough for the tart shells. Add the salt, cinnamon, nutmeg, almond, and dates into the food processor.
2. Pulse this until it becomes crumbly and then continue to blend until you get a sticky ball to form.
3. Take these out of the food processor and use the dough to make 8 balls that are equal in size.

4. Press these into a mini muffin pan, and then let it set in the fridge for about ten minutes before taking them out to use.

5. After cleaning out the food processor, combine all of the ingredients for the filling inside until they are smooth.

6. To each of the shells that you made, add in the filling. Top with a raspberry before serving.

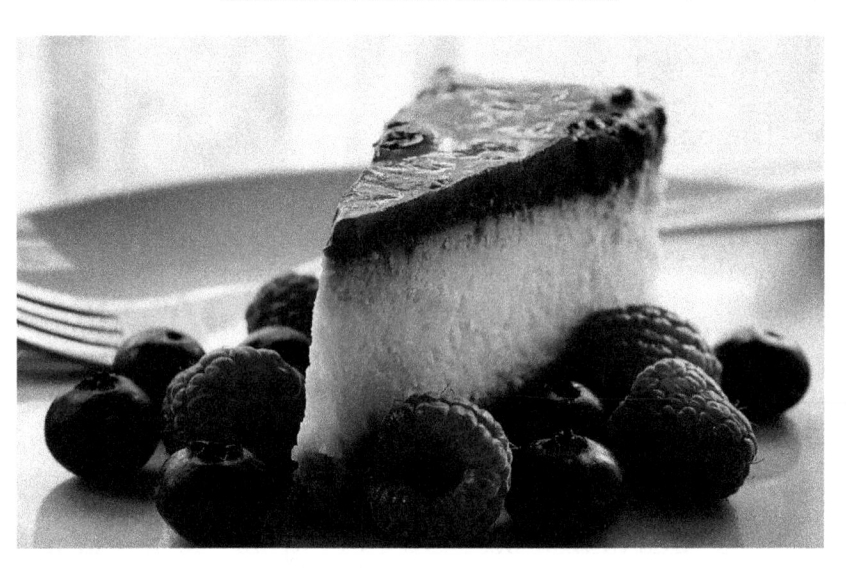

Chocolate Donut Holes

What's inside:

- Cinnamon (.25 tsp.)

- Vanilla (.5 tsp.)

- Raw honey (.25 tsp.)

- Cacao powder (.25 c.)
- Salt (.25 tsp.)
- Coconut oil (.5 Tbsp.)
- Drained dates (10)
- Raw almonds (.5 c.)
- Raw walnuts (.5 c.)

How to make:

1. To start this recipe, take out a food processor and add the almonds and walnuts inside until finely ground.
2. Add the dates to this mixture and process for another two minutes until well combined.
3. Now, you can add in the rest of the ingredients as well, combining until nice and smooth.
4. Take the dough and roll it into small balls. Add to the fridge and let these chill for a minimum of a few hours before serving.

Banana and Oatmeal Cookies

What's inside:

- Salt (.25 tsp.)
- Ground cloves (.25 tsp.)
- Nutmeg (.25 tsp.)
- Cinnamon (.25 tsp.)
- Raisins (.25 c.)
- Rolled oats (.5 c.)
- Mashed bananas (1)

How to make:

1. Turn on the oven and let it heat up to 350 degrees. While the oven is preparing, take out a baking sheet and line it with some parchment paper.
2. Bring out a bowl and combine together all of the ingredients until smooth. Drop a bit of this mixture onto your prepared baking tray and then place in the oven.
3. After 15 minutes, the cookies should be lightly browned, and you can take them out of the oven. Give them time to cool down before serving.

Cinnamon Buns

What's inside:

- Melted coconut butter (.5 Tbsp.)
- Coconut cream (1 Tbsp.)
- Raw honey (1 Tbsp.)
- Almonds (.25 c.)
- Nutmeg (1 tsp.)
- Cinnamon (3 Tbsp.)
- Salt (.25 tsp.)
- Vanilla (1 tsp.)
- Pitted dates (1.5 c.)
- Walnuts (.5 c.)
- Almonds (1.5 c.)

How to make:

1. Bring out the food processor and pulse together the walnuts and almonds until you get fine flour. Then add in the salt, vanilla, and dates and pulse to combine.
2. Take out half the mixture and set to the side. Then add in the nutmeg and cinnamon to the food processor and pulse to combine.

3. Take out the dough and then roll out each half of the dough (the part in the food processor and the part you took out), into rectangles that are the same size.

4. Top the regular dough with .25 of the slivered almonds. Place the cinnamon and nutmeg dough over the other dough and press down. Top with the rest of the almonds.

5. Roll this dough up to form a bit log. Wrap in parchment paper and add to the freezer for 60 minutes or more.

6. While these chill, you can work on making the glaze. To do this, bring out a bowl and combine the coconut butter, coconut cream, and honey together.

7. After 60 minutes, take the cinnamon roll out and slice it into even slices. Drizzle the glaze on top and then enjoy.

Bonus

Understanding the Use of Herbs in the Alkaline Diet

When you choose to go on the alkaline diet plan, you will find that there are a lot of recipes that are going to ask you to bring in some herbs. These are great to use because they are simple, they add a lot of flavoring to your meals, and they are not going to cause you to get sick or have to worry about added acid in your diet like dressings, sugars, and more are. In fact, when you take a look back through some of the different recipes that we have gone through with the previous chapters, you will notice that a lot of them rely heavily on herbs and other spices to help keep us healthy.

That is where this chapter is going to start off with. We are going to look at some of the most popular herbs that work well with the alkaline diet. Adding these into the diet often, and mixing them up can ensure that you are going to get as much flavoring into the diet plan as possible. Some of the best herbs that are approved on the alkaline diet and can help to improve your health overall will include the following:

Basil

You will find that it is very hard and pretty much impossible for disease to survive when the body has an alkaline environment.

Instead, this disease is going to do the best when the environment is more acidic. And this is why almost all kinds of diseases are going to begin with a form of inflammation in some parts of the body. This is where basil is going to come into play.

Basil, which is often known as the king of herbs, is one that is able to fight off inflammation. This is because it has a ton of oils inside of it that are not just anti-bacterial and anti-aging, but they can also help to fight off some of the inflammation inside. Basil is easy to add into some of your tomato-based soups and dishes that have tomatoes, making the dish pop with flavor without having to put in flavorings that are going to cause you some harm.

Cilantro

If you are already a fan of cilantro, then this one needs to become a staple in your pantry. This is going to come in low in calories, and it has a lot of the nutrients that are essential to keeping you full, stopping you from eating a lot of empty calories, and helping with the various metabolic processes that are found with your body. In addition, it is going to be high in some of the vitamins that your body needs, including Vitamin A, C, and K.

In addition to some of the antioxidant and anti-inflammatory properties that are found inside, you will find that this herb is going to taste really good in a lot of the foods that you are enjoying. From the stems to the leaves to the seeds and more, you are sure to find plenty of uses for adding cilantro to your meal plan.

Cinnamon

For desserts, snacks, breakfasts, and even some main meals, you will find that nothing is better than adding in some cinnamon to the foods that you are eating. Add in that this herb is going to be good for helping with diabetes while reducing inflammation and the acidity of your diet, and you know cinnamon is one of the best choices for your needs.

In one study that was published in the American Journal of Clinical Nutrition in 2007, it was found that in subjects who were healthy, consuming about 6 grams of cinnamon was able to reduce their glucose response when they were done with a meal. There have also been other studies that show how cinnamon is able to lower total cholesterol, LDL, and triglycerides in those who suffer from type 2 diabetes.

Ginger

Another herb that we need to take a look at is ginger. This is a powerful aid to digestion and an antimicrobial herb. Ginger root is going to be really potent, containing phenolic compounds that help us to digest our food better while also maintaining the tone of the intestinal muscles and neutralizing excess acidity that is in the stomach without irritating the abdomen.

For the most part, people are going to use ginger to help with pain and as an agent to stop inflammation. This is why it is often recommended when it is time to work with allergies, respiratory issues, chronic muscular pains, and to treat arthritis. In one article that was published in 2005 from the Journal of Medicinal Food, it was discovered that the consumption of ginger is able to modulate the biochemical pathways that are related to chronic inflammation. In addition, there are other studies that show how ginger is able to help with migraine headaches, motion sickness, and nausea related to pregnancy.

Peppermint

No look at herbs is going to be complete without taking a look at peppermint. This herb is going to go way beyond some of the flavoring that you get, whether you add it on topically or you consume it. It is going to have a lot of benefits thanks to some of the main ingredients, including menthone and menthol. There are a lot of different uses for peppermint, including helping with IBS, a remedy for colic, and as a digestive aid.

Researchers from Germany have found that when taken among subjects who are healthy, the oil from peppermint can help to slow down the transit time of food in the small intestine, can be relaxing to the gallbladder, and can help aid the digestion in the stomach. And since it is higher in dietary fiber for being an herb, it is considered a must when we look at a weight loss plan. Adding a few leaves of peppermint to a salad or to some other dish, even dessert, will be just what is needed to help keep you healthy as possible.

Oregano

The next option on the list is going to be oregano. This one has been used in the past as an anti-fungal and anti-microbial agent, but it is going to be full of a lot of other nutrients as well. Since it is full of potassium, calcium, magnesium, iron, Vitamins A and C, copper, beta carotene, and more, this is definitely something that you need to add into your diet.

Rosemary

If you are looking to go with an herb that is going to help provide you with the antioxidants you need to release some of the toxins in your body, then rosemary is the answer that you are looking for. This herb was once thought to be the thing you needed to ward off any bad influences in your life, but it could be used to help detox the body, lose weight, and fight off the inflammation.

One study that was published in 2006 out of Finland has even suggested that some of the compounds found in rosemary are able to counteract some of the harmful oxidation that we often see when heating up extra virgin olive oil. Add in that it contains a ton of mineral manganese and vitamin C, and you have a great herb to help keep you healthy.

Thyme

Whether you are making a French-based dish or just looking to find another alkaline diet-friendly herb to add to the mix, thyme is definitely your friend here. Thyme is going to help boost up your immune system thanks to the fact that it is loaded with vitamins C and A. Researchers from the University of Brighton, East Sussex were able to find that thyme oil was actually effective when it came to killing MRSA, or methicillin-resistant Staph auereas, which is usually going to be resistant to some other antibiotics that are tried. Add in some healthy B-vitamins to the mix, and you are going to see some great results in the process.

Thyme is going to be great in lots of stews and any kind of braised recipes that you want to try. You can also work on adding them to vegetables before roasting them or throw into a marinade that you use on poultry, especially if that recipe is supposed to have garlic and or lemon in it. Or, scrambled eggs go well with the thyme herb as well.

These are just some of the herbs that you need to consider adding into your diet when you go on the alkaline diet. There are a lot of choices that you are able to make with herbs and spices, and many of them are not only going to be able to make your meals taste better, they are also going to help improve your health in many different manners, just like we talked about earlier. When you are ready to get the most out of the alkaline diet, make sure to check out some of these herbs and find out different ways that you can start adding them to your meals today.

Conclusion

Thank you for making it through to the end of *Alkaline Diet Cookbook*. Let's hope it was informative and able to provide you with all of the tools you need to achieve your goals whatever they may be.

The next step is to start implementing the alkaline diet into your lifestyle. The alkaline diet is going to be a great choice to help you get your pH levels in check while helping you to lose weight, fight off disease and inflammation, and so much more. We have spent some time learning more about this kind of diet plan, and how it is able to benefit you and give you the good health that you are looking for in your life.

From learning about the alkaline diet to seeing some of the many health benefits that come with this plan and more, we have spent a lot of time learning about the alkaline diet and what it is all about. We also looked at some of the best means and recipes that you are able to work with in order to see results from this diet plan as a beginner.

When you are ready to learn a bit more about the alkaline diet and what it is able to do for you, make sure to check out this diet plan to help you get started, and get in your best health ever.

Finally, if you found this book useful in any way, a review on Amazon is always appreciated!

CPSIA information can be obtained
at www.ICGtesting.com
Printed in the USA
LVHW010133220221
679513LV00002B/71